Evis Sala · Alan H. Freeman ·
David J. Lomas · Helmut Ringl

# Radiology for Surgeons in Clinical Practice

Foreword by Johannes Zacherl

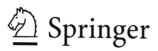

Springer

Evis Sala
Department of Radiology
Addenbrooke's Hospital
Cambridge
UK

Alan H. Freeman
Department of Radiology
Addenbrooke's Hospital
Cambridge
UK

David J. Lomas
Department of Radiology
Addenbrooke's Hospital
Cambridge
UK

Helmut Ringl
Department of Radiology
Medical University Vienna
Vienna
Austria

ISBN: 978-1-84800-095-7     e-ISBN: 978-1-84800-096-4
DOI: 10.1007/978-1-84800-096-4

British Library Cataloguing in Publication Data
Radiology for surgeons in clinical practice
   1. Interventional radiology  2. Diagnosis, Surgical
   I. Sala, Evis
   616′ .0757
ISBN-13: 9781848000957

Library of Congress Control Number: 2007943248

Springer Science+Business Media
springer.com

# Foreword

In the daily medical routine, recent refinements of several modern imaging techniques enable us to enhance diagnostic accuracy. Tremendous efforts in radiology have been made to help us to avoid inappropriate interventions and treatments by a misleading diagnosis and to obviate false-negative results, too.

The rapid development of imaging techniques requires continuing theoretical updating in this field by publications like the current compendium. Theoretical principles of radiology methods are brought up in a concise manner, and according to the composition of modern medical university curricula, the pathology findings are arranged and described in dependence on clinical symptoms rather than as a listing of diseases. This configuration therefore turns the opus in front of you into a useful and valuable companion during surgical education. The initial tentativeness of young trainees and of the nonradiology "old hand" in the face of modern imaging techniques and new contrast agents, will rapidly disappear and turn into enlightened familiarity, helping one to use those fine arts in discovering the patient's problem and in the planning of treatment strategy.

In the era of interdisciplinary boards and discussion, surgeons traditionally are an essential driving force. This position demands an expertise in imaging, which may be strengthened by a special advantage: the surgeon is in the unique position to immediately compare radiology findings with the intracorporeal situation during surgery, what we often might call "the clinical truth." This circumstance allows for an accurate learning effect, which should be a central aspect of training in clinical decision making. A further advantage of close-to-the-patient disciplines is the correlation between clinical signs and radiology findings. I do not want to end this foreword without emphasizing the need of keeping an eye on the clinical signals and additionally on information delivered by modern technology.

My first mentor repeated the claim that "the surgeon is the better radiologist." Thanks to the authors of this book, this sentence may again become true.

Johannes Zacherl

# Preface

Hamilton Bailey, in his time perhaps the foremost teacher of surgery in the English language, described assessment of the acute abdomen in his book, *Demonstration of Physical Signs in Clinical Surgery* (1960), as follows:

> Physical signs and their interpretation reach a high pinnacle of importance in the diagnosis of acute abdominal disease. Frequently an urgent and all important diagnosis has to be formulated by their aid alone.

How times have changed and the perspective from nearly half a century later is completely different.

The history and clinical examination still remain the bedrock of diagnosis but virtually no patient today will pass through the hands of a surgeon without some form of radiological imaging, from the simple plain radiographic image to complex 3D reformats of data sets acquired during CT and MR examinations. In this context, diagnostic imaging has revolutionized the way surgery is practiced. It thus behooves the surgical trainee to remain abreast of all the techniques available and to be cognizant of their advantages and disadvantages.

In this small book, the authors – all radiologists – have attempted to look at the patient from the clinical perspective of symptoms and signs, and then to formulate the relevant imaging which would be appropriate for their management.

Our intention has been to produce a radiological guide for the surgical trainee, without delving too deeply into the technological processes of image acquisition and manipulation. We hope it helps.

Our particular thanks go to Melissa Morton of Springer UK for the encouragement to produce this book and to Barbara Chernow and all the production team at Springer who have been responsible for bringing it to fruition.

Evis Sala
Alan H. Freeman
David J. Lomas
Helmut Ringl

# Contents

# Part I
## Principles of Imaging

Imaging investigations are an essential part of the management of patients presenting with surgical problems. To have a logical plan of investigation for a particular clinical situation, an understanding of the imaging techniques is required including the method of generating an image, costs, strengths, weaknesses, and associated risks. This chapter introduces the basic concepts of the available imaging modalities and their advantages and disadvantages in clinical practice.

## 1.1 Plain Radiographs, or X-rays

X-rays are electromagnetic radiation with an energy and frequency substantially greater than visible light. They are generated within an X-ray tube, in which electrons are accelerated at a small metal target from which X-rays are then emitted. These are then collimated into a shaped beam and directed at the relevant part of a patient. Depending upon the intervening tissue's attenuation properties, a characteristic pattern of X-rays is transmitted through the imaged part. Conventionally, these X-rays are then converted by phosphor screens into light photons, which expose photographic film subsequently processed to create the *X-ray film* or *radiograph* viewed on a lightbox. Increasingly, these systems are being replaced by solid-state X-ray detectors (e.g., selenium-based or amorphous silicon–based materials), which convert X-rays indirectly (computed radiography; CR) or directly (direct radiography; DR) into electrical signals, providing digital and *filmless* acquisition. These are usually reviewed on workstations but can be converted to film if needed. Image contrast relies on the fact that different parts of the body attenuate (stop) X-rays better than others. Lungs are mostly gas, and most X-rays pass straight through, whereas bones are high in calcium, which absorbs X-rays to a high degree. A tissue structure is often only visible if it lies adjacent to another tissue of different density. In general terms, the major attenuation differences occur between gas, soft tissues, fat, and bone. Therefore, radiographic examinations are particularly good for directly imaging bony structures and those containing gas, such as the lungs. Conventional radiographs are *projection* techniques providing no intrinsic *depth* information, therefore interpreting abdominal and pelvic examinations requires some skill, for example to understand the patterns of normal and abnormal gas and fluid distribution.

An additional feature of X-rays is that they may be used to obtain dynamic information using an image intensifier. This is termed *fluoroscopy* and allows real-time observation during a range of diagnostic and therapeutic procedures. Despite newer, more sophisticated forms of imaging, a plain radiograph remains one of the cheapest, fastest, and simplest ways of detecting many problems; however, they lack sensitivity and specificity. The diagnostic advantage of the use of X-rays typically outweighs the risks from the effects of ionizing radiation (see Section 1.3.2).

| *Advantages* | *Disadvantages* |
|---|---|
| • Fast | • Uses ionizing radiation |
| • Relatively inexpensive | • Limited soft tissue contrast |
| • High spatial resolution | • Projection method lacking any true depth discrimination |
| • Widely available | |

# 1.2 Contrast Medium Studies

A limitation of plain X-ray examination is that most of the soft tissue structures of the body are of similar radiographic density. To visualize these various soft tissue structures, contrast agents were developed and improved during the 20th century. Although negative contrast using gas was widely used, most studies now employ positive contrast media that attenuate X-rays by means of their high atomic number. These agents include barium sulfate used mainly in the gastrointestinal tract and water-soluble agents containing bound iodine that may also be used intravenously.

## 1.2.1 Oral Contrast Medium Studies

Barium sulfate is an inert, insoluble substance that can be taken orally and used to outline the various portions of the gastrointestinal tract. Improved results and higher sensitivity are achieved with *double-contrast* studies combining both gas distension and barium coating of the luminal surface of the organ being examined.

An important issue is the choice of contrast media in case of suspected esophageal tear or gastrointestinal perforation. Barium in the mediastinal or peritoneal cavity is harmful and may cause mediastinal or peritoneal fibrosis. Water-soluble non-ionic contrast media are safer, although they lack the level of anatomic definition created by barium. Similarly, if aspiration is suspected or likely, water-soluble, non-ionic contrast media should always be used first, followed by barium if there is no obvious leak. Ionic, water-soluble contrast media such as Gastrografin (Schering Health Care Ltd., Burgess Hill, West Sussex, UK) should be avoided as they cause severe pulmonary edema if aspirated.

Examples of barium studies are as follows:

*Barium swallow*: This is used for the imaging of the pharynx and the esophagus. It is one of the first-line investigation methods for esophageal disorders, particularly in cases of dysphagia. Good fluoroscopy is important, and video recordings are made as the barium is swallowed if a motility disorder is suspected.

*Barium meal:* Used for examination of the lower esophagus, stomach, and duodenum. Double-contrast techniques provide excellent detail of the mucosal surface of the stomach and duodenum. Although considered the basic technique for radiologic investigation of the stomach, it has been largely replaced by endoscopy.

*Small bowel study:* Used to examine the structure and motility of the small bowel. Barium can be given either orally (barium *follow-through*) or administered via a tube placed into the distal duodenum or proximal jejunum (small bowel enema or enteroclysis). Barium introduced directly into the small bowel offers exquisite visualization by creating an uninterrupted column of contrast medium distending the jejunum and ileum. This facilitates detection of any structural abnormality that might be present. Capsule endoscopy has replaced this technique for subtle lesions with no morphologic changes (e.g., some arterio-vascular malformations).

*Barium enema:* Double contrast using barium and air via a rectal tube to outline the lumen and mucosa of the large bowel. Despite the increasing role of colonoscopy, double-contrast barium enema remains widely used for examination of the large bowel. Limited single-contrast studies can be used to demonstrate and confirm the level of a colonic obstruction or a fistula.

## *1.2.2 Intravenous Contrast Medium Studies*

Intravenous contrast medium is used to enhance vessel and tissue contrast in various X-ray–dependent imaging modalities. After intravenous administration, the contrast agent passes through the venous and arterial system, thus rendering these vessels visible. During circulation, a certain amount of the contrast medium passes through the vessel wall and distributes to the extracellular fluid of the surrounding tissue/organs producing the necessary contrast to show anatomic and pathologic details. The contrast medium is then excreted through the kidneys and finally delineates the urinary tract.

Intravenous contrast media that are used for X-ray examinations are based on iodine. They can be categorized as ionic and non-ionic, depending on their molecular structure and osmotic behavior in the blood. Non-ionic contrast media such as Iopamidol (Bracco UK Ltd., Wooburn Green, Buckinghamshire, UK) have less risk of adverse reactions (in part related to their low osmolarity) but are typically more expensive than their ionic equivalents. Side effects include nephrotoxicity and allergic reactions ranging from mild skin alterations to anaphylaxis. Therefore, elevated serum creatinine levels and a previous history of contrast medium allergy represent relative contraindications, and an alternative imaging modality such as ultrasound (US) or magnetic resonance imaging (MRI) should be considered. If the use of an iodine-based contrast medium is unavoidable, high-risk patients should receive a premedication with corticosteroids (prednisolone 30 mg orally 12 and 2 hours before contrast medium) and antihistamines. To reduce nephrotoxicity, all patients should be adequately hydrated before the contrast medium injection, and intravenous fluids may be needed for those with known renal impairment.

## 1.2.2.1 Intravenous Urography

Intravenous urography (IVU) is used to investigate urinary tract disorders, especially renal colic. It provides some anatomic and functional renal information but is most useful for demonstrating the ureters and pelvicaliceal systems 5 to 20 minutes after injection of intravenous contrast medium. An initial plain radiograph (to look for renal tract calcification) is always obtained. In the case of acute renal colic, IVU has been partially replaced by low-dose unenhanced computed tomography (CT) in many institutions. The latter yields not only higher sensitivity and specificity but offers also additional information of all other abdominal organs.

## 1.2.2.2 X-ray Angiography

*Arteriography* demonstrates narrowing or obstruction (by plaque, thrombus, or embolus) of major organ arteries such as the coronary, cerebral, or carotid. It is achieved by injection of contrast medium directly into the artery via a catheter. This relatively invasive technique also allows therapeutic interventions such as dilating narrowed arteries (angioplasty) or blocking off leaking or ruptured vessels (embolization). The development of less invasive techniques such as Doppler ultrasound, computed tomography angiography (CTA), and magnetic resonance angiography (MRA) has replaced the majority of diagnostic angiography.

The most common approach for both diagnostic and therapeutic angiography is via direct puncture of the common femoral artery. Other approaches can be used when the femoral approach is impossible because of occlusive iliac disease. Different catheter sizes and shapes are used for particular procedures such as selective arteriography of celiac axis and mesenteric and renal arteries. These techniques are invasive with small but definite associated risks including accidental rupture or blockage of a vessel, which may occasionally lead to serious morbidity or mortality.

*Digital subtraction angiography* takes advantage of digital data acquisition, storage, and processing. First, an image is taken without contrast medium in the vessel: the *mask*. Then images are taken as contrast medium is being injected: the *contrast film*. Finally, the computer subtracts the mask from the contrast film leaving an image of the vessels without the background bone. This technique offers superior contrast resolution with lower doses of contrast medium, though the spatial resolution is inferior to conventional angiography. It plays an important role in interventional studies as the images can be viewed immediately.

In *venography*, contrast medium is injected via a needle or catheter positioned directly into the vein to be imaged, and series of plain radiographs/digital images are taken. The role of venography in occlusive disease of the leg veins has been largely superseded by compression ultrasound.

# 1.3 Cross-sectional Imaging

## 1.3.1 Ultrasound

US provides real-time cross-sectional imaging of soft tissues. Because of its ability to differentiate tissue characteristics and demonstrate blood flow, US has become a valuable technique for evaluating solid organs and vessels as well as an excellent method of guiding interventional procedures. US is a relatively inexpensive, rapid imaging modality that avoids ionizing radiation. It is patient friendly, as it often requires no special preparation. Mobile US machines can be taken to the bedside or into the operating theater, providing a great advantage for emergency use. US can also be used to guide tissue biopsy or drainage procedures because of the interactive nature of real-time US.

US uses high-frequency sound waves produced by piezo-electric crystals that transform electrical energy into longitudinal compression waves (2 to 20 MHz); these echoes are reflected echoes in a similar fashion to sonar and radar. Modern systems use pulses of US and by timing the delay for the echoes to return calculate the depth at which the reflected echo originated. Sophisticated computing, crystal multiplexing, and signal processing allows for real-time image display.

Image contrast is generated by tissues that have varying *acoustic impedance*, and at cellular and tissue interfaces, impedance mismatches result in varying amounts of echo reflection. The terms increased or decreased *echoreflectivity* are used to describe tissues appearing bright or dark, respectively. Pure fluid reflects no sound and is often termed *anechoic*, typically appearing black on an image.

A major limitation of ultrasound imaging is the inability to see through gas and bone, limiting particularly the examination of the iliac fossae and retroperitoneum. Endoluminal transducers can also be used to avoid problems with obscuring gas and to improve resolution; for example, transvaginal, transrectal, endoscopic, intraductal (biliary and pancreatic), and intravascular transducers have all been developed.

*Doppler US* is based on the *Doppler effect*. When the object reflecting US waves is moving, it shifts the frequency of the returning echoes, creating a higher frequency if it is moving toward the probe and a lower frequency if it is moving away from the probe. The frequency shift is directly related to the object's velocity allowing a real-time display of estimated blood velocity, which can be useful in large vessels to estimate stenoses (e.g., for the carotid and cardiac valves). This information can be graphed against time (duplex US and M-mode) or used to provide a color overlay on a real-time image (color Doppler imaging).

*Contrast agents* have recently been developed using small "microbubbles" able to pass through the capillary bed and provide increased echoreflectivity. Clinical applications being evaluated include fallopian tube patency, detection of vesico-ureteric reflux, assessment of portal venous patency in cirrhosis, diagnosis of renal artery stenosis, and so forth. Recently, liver specific microbubbles have been developed to increase sensitivity in the detection of focal liver malignancies.

US is considered a very safe technique, and is widely used in pediatrics and obstetrics. There are theoretical concerns related to tissue heating and cavitation within cells that limit the power used, particularly using endovaginal probes in early pregnancy.

| *Advantages* | *Disadvantages* |
|---|---|
| • Cheap | • Cannot see through gas or bone |
| • Portable | • Limited window and filmed record |
| • Safe | • More operator dependent than CT |

## 1.3.2 Computed Tomography

CT uses X-rays to obtain cross-sectional images that provide depth information. Modern systems can rapidly and robustly image a combination of soft tissue, bone, and blood vessels.

The use of a calibrated X-ray detector system provides much improved soft tissue contrast compared with conventional radiographs although the mechanism of image contrast remains the same. CT is increasingly used in both acute and chronically ill patients and is also essential to guide percutaneous interventional procedures such as biopsies and drainage of fluid collections.

Current CT systems use continuous spiral data acquisition in the axial plane as the patient moves through a rotating fan-beam of X-rays. A volume of data is acquired that may be reformatted in other anatomic planes as required. Intravenous contrast medium allows for vascular imaging and also improved organ imaging with the detection of pathologic lesions as based on their vascular enhancement. Owing to the short total acquisition time of spiral CT, different contrast enhancement phases are now possible. These multiphase studies can further improve the characterization of focal lesions. *Multislice* spiral CT scanners can simultaneously collect up to 64 or more slices of data during each spiral rotation reducing examination times and allowing improved image reformatting.

CT is particularly sensitive for detecting acute hemorrhage, gas, and calcium and for these reasons is widely used in the evaluation of acute trauma. Other recent applications of CT include use as a first-line investigation in the diagnosis of abdominal pain, appendicitis, and renal colic. CT examination is fast and simple, enabling a quick overview of possible life-threatening pathology, and facilitates a dedicated surgical treatment.

As a result of all these new applications and improvements, there has been a dramatic increase in the number of CT examinations, which now account for the majority of medical irradiation of the population. As a result of this ionizing radiation, there is an estimated increased lifetime risk of 1 in 2500 solid malignancies from the dose of a single routine abdomen-pelvic CT. Therefore, it is important that the use of CT is managed appropriately by clinicians and radiologists to ensure that CT is the appropriate investigation in a given clinical situation rather than other "safer" techniques such as US or MRI.

## 1.3.3 Magnetic Resonance Imaging

MRI provides multiplanar imaging of the body with excellent soft tissue discrimination and a range of contrast mechanisms. Historically, relatively long imaging times made magnetic resonance (MR) less robust for imaging the abdomen and pelvis although new fast-imaging techniques are now available. It has the particular advantage of avoiding the use of ionizing radiation.

MRI exploits the ability of nuclei with an uneven number of nuclei to resonate (at specific frequencies) between energy states in a magnetic field. As approximately 70% of the human body is composed of water and fat, protons are the primary nucleus used for imaging. When placed in a strong magnetic field, the protons resonate at a particular frequency and reach equilibrium. This equilibrium can be disturbed by a radiofrequency-pulse *excitation* and the return to equilibrium observed and used to generate images. *T1 and T2 relaxation times* are decay constants reflecting the ability of nuclei to return to equilibrium after excitation. Different tissues have varying T1 and T2 properties that allow them to be discriminated in an image. The spatial localization of the tissues within the image is complicated and relies on the mathematical Fourier transform and additional transiently applied magnetic fields.

Soft tissue contrast is superior to X-ray–based CT imaging and readily allows separation of liver, spleen, muscle, fat, tendons, cartilage, and blood flow; however, the ability to discriminate between calcium, air, and dense fibrous tissue is limited, as these materials all lack protons and therefore generate no signal. MR can generate angiograms (MRA) utilizing both intrinsic flow and intravenous bolus injections of contrast medium (relying on T1 shortening for the vascular signal). In addition, heavily T2-weighted (T2W) images using intrinsic fluids (that have a long T2 value) as contrast have been used to noninvasively demonstrate the biliary tree, avoiding the need for invasive endoscopic retrograde cholangiopancreatography (ERCP) examinations.

MRI has quickly evolved in recent years to become the primary diagnostic imaging technique for many neurologic and musculoskeletal problems. It is used selectively in abdomen and pelvis, for example in staging pelvic malignancy, mapping perineal fistulae, and detecting common bile duct stones. It plays an important role in preoperative staging of tumors of the rectum, prostate, ovary, and uterus. MRA is replacing many conventional diagnostic angiographic procedures, for example in the diagnosis of renal artery stenosis and the preoperative evaluation of kidney transplant donors.

MR contrast agents are based around gadolinium chelates, which are administered intravenously and operate in a similar fashion to the iodinated agents used in CT. They are not organ or pathology specific but may be valuable in distinguishing tumor recurrence from changes due to previous surgery. Recently, gadolinium-based contrast media have been associated with a serious and rare systemic fibrosing condition. The condition appears to be limited to patients with preexisting severe renal impairment, and in such patients caution should be exercised when using these agents. *Blood-pool* and *liver-specific* contrast agents have been developed that allow more prolonged investigation time and increase the conspicuity of liver lesions. There is ongoing research in the development of tumor-specific and targeted agents such as necrosis-specific and inflammation-specific agents. Although not commonly used in clinical practice, several studies have proved MR useful in assisting interventional procedures such as biopsy guidance and to monitor radiofrequency, cryoablation, and laser therapies.

MRI is a relatively safe technique although the use of a strong magnetic field may damage pacemakers and cause metal fragments in the retina or brain to move, so patients are routinely screened for these and other risks. Surgical clips and joint replacements are, however, not usually a risk to the patient although they may degrade the images. MRI is also relatively motion sensitive leading to image artifacts. This is one reason why MRI has been less robust for imaging acutely ill patients when compared with CT.

| *Advantages* | *Disadvantages* |
|---|---|
| • Excellent soft tissue contrast<br>• Multiplanar acquisition | • Complex to understand and interpret<br>• Motion sensitive |

## 1.4 Nuclear Medicine Imaging

Nuclear medicine (NM) provides primarily functional rather than anatomic imaging and relies on detecting emitted gamma rays from radiopharmaceuticals administered to patients. This *functional information* allows NM techniques to diagnose certain diseases earlier than other techniques that provide mainly anatomic information. For example, bone infection results in increased cellular activity of bone, causing radionuclides to be taken up in greater amounts by infected bone. NM techniques may demonstrate this change earlier than the anatomic image provided by a plain radiograph or CT examination. The amount of radiation that is taken up and then emitted by a specific body part is linked to the metabolic activity and cellular function of the organ or tissue.

NM studies are typically performed using radiation detectors or *gamma cameras* after the oral or intravenous introduction of radioactive chemicals (radionuclides, radio-pharmaceuticals, or radiotracers that emit gamma rays) into the body. Radiopharmaceuticals are usually formulated to localize in the specific part of the body to be studied. The radionuclide substances used in NM imaging are either synthesized radioactive substances, such as technetium, or radioactive forms of elements that are naturally found in the body, such as iodine. The emitted gamma rays are detected by the gamma camera using a large crystal detector and are spatially localized. The gamma rays are then converted into light and subsequent electrical signal, which is used to create the image. As the method relies on the emission of gamma rays, the achievable spatial resolution is relatively low compared with other techniques, but this is compensated for by the additional functional information.

*Emission computed tomography (ECT)* is a method of obtaining three-dimensional localization of the radionuclide within the patient. ECT involves cross-sectional data acquisition and reconstruction similar to CT. It can be achieved by *single positron emission computed tomography (SPECT)* and *positron emission tomography (PET)*. SPECT is based on the detection of single gamma rays emitted from radionuclides such as technetium-99m and thalium-201. SPECT images represent uptake measured from different angular views around the patient so they can be reconstructed in different anatomic planes. PET involves coincident detection of paired high-energy photons emitted simultaneously after the annihilation of positron-emitting radionuclides such as carbon-11, fluorine-18, and so forth. PET is becoming increasingly important in oncology, being able to differentiate in certain situations between active tumor growth and necrotic tissue. PET is more sensitive than SPECT, but PET scanners are much more costly than SPECT scanners and are often only available in the largest medical centers.

| *Advantages* | *Disadvantages* |
| --- | --- |
| • Provides functional information | • Poor anatomic definition |
| • Detection of radiographically occult abnormalities | • Not readily available in emergency situations |

To overcome the low spatial resolution and the lack of anatomic detail, PET-CT was recently introduced. It combines the anatomic information of CT and the metabolic information provided by PET. This ability to demonstrate abnormal metabolic activity enables PET-CT to differentiate benign from malign tissue (e.g., a scar from a neoplasm).

# *Suggestions for Further Reading*

1. Harvey CJ, Pilcher JM, Eckersley RJ, Blomley MJK, Cosgrove DO. Advances in ultrasound. Clin Radiol 2002;57:157–177.
2. Klingenbeck–Regn K, Schaller S, Flohr T, Ohnesorge B, Kopp A, Baum U. Subsecond multi-slice computed tomography: basics and applications. Eur J Radiol 1999;31:110–124.
3. Terrier F, Grossholz M, Becker CD (eds). Spiral CT of the abdomen. Springer, Berlin, 2002.
4. McRobbie DW, Moore E, Graves MJ, Prince MR. MRI from picture to proton. Cambridge University Press, Cambridge, UK, 2003.
5. Murray IPC, Ell PJ (eds). Nuclear medicine in clinical diagnosis and treatment. Churchill Livingstone, Edinburgh, 1994.
6. Hart B, Wall BF. Radiation exposure of the UK population from the medical and dental x-ray examinations. NRPB, March 2002. NRPB. Document W4 pp 1–41. National Radiation Protection Board Health Protection Agency. Chilton; Didcot, Oxford, UK.
7. Thomsen HS, Morcos SK, ESUR. ESUR guidelines on contrast media. Abdom Imaging 2006;31(2):131–140.
8. Heneghan JP, McGuire KA, Leder RA, DeLong DM, Yoshizumi T, Nelson RC. Helical CT for nephrolithiasis and ureterolithiasis: comparison of conventional and reduced radiation-dose techniques. Radiology 2003;229(2):575–580.
9. Kapoor V, McCook BM, Torok FS. An introduction to PET-CT imaging. Radiographics 2004;24(2):523–543.

# Part II
## Imaging of Common Clinical Problems

As has been seen, radiology plays an increasingly important role in the management of the surgical patient, both for preoperative diagnosis and postoperative management. Techniques have evolved rapidly since the discovery of X-rays in 1895, and the availability and combination of different imaging modalities have improved the ability to achieve rapid and accurate diagnoses. Image guidance allows the use of percutaneous procedures, such as tumor biopsy and abscess drainage, which avoid the need for open surgery. Radiographic studies remain the first-line imaging technique in many clinical situations although cross-sectional imaging with ultrasound (US), magnetic resonance imaging (MRI), and especially computed tomography (CT) are now widely used in patients with acute abdominal pain and after trauma. The aim of this chapter is to provide a simple diagnostic framework for common surgical situations.

## 2.1 Pain and the Acute Abdomen

Most diseases of thoracic and abdominal viscera are associated with pain at some time during their course. This section focuses on imaging of certain common clinical situations where pain is a prominent symptom.

# 2.1.1 Chest Pain

It is important for the surgeon to recognize certain imaging features of pathologies resulting in chest pain although physicians rather than surgeons will most commonly deal with nontraumatic chest pain.

## 2.1.1.1 Pneumothorax

Pneumothorax reflects the accumulation of air in the pleural space and commonly presents with pleuritic chest pain and/or dyspnea. Diagnosis of pneumothorax is made with a chest radiograph, which may also demonstrate complications and relevant underlying lung pathology. Signs indicating a pneumothorax on an erect chest radiograph include:

- Visceral pleural line separated from the chest wall by a transradiant area devoid of blood vessels
- Deep costophrenic sulcus laterally
- Visible anterior costophrenic recess (*double-diaphragm* sign)
- Increased transradiancy of ipsilateral lung or hypochondrium
- Ipsilateral depression of the diaphragm
- Contralateral mediastinal shift

The last two signs in combination and particularly mediastinal shift indicate a tension pneumothorax that typically causes rapid deterioration in a patient's clinical condition and requires prompt intervention. In situations when an erect inspiratory chest radiograph is indeterminate, an expiratory or lateral decubitus radiograph may help in making the diagnosis. Occasionally, it is difficult to differentiate pneumothorax from other pulmonary lesions

FIGURE 2.1.1.1A,B. Pneumothorax. (A) In this erect chest radiograph (CXR), the visceral pleural line (arrow) is separated from the chest wall by a transradiant area lacking in vascular markings indicating a right pneumothorax. (B) Left-sided pneumothorax (arrows) causing mild mediastinal shift to the right.

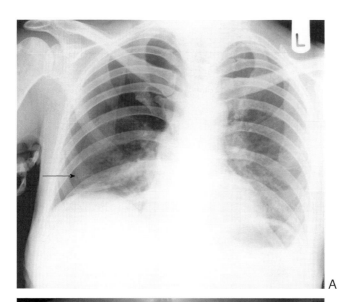

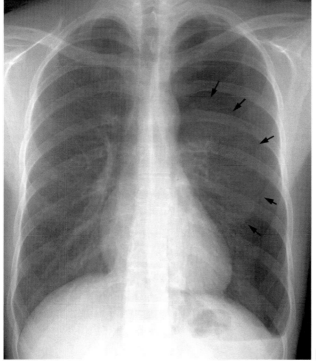

or overlying transradiancies such as simple cysts, emphysematous bullae, pneumatoceles, pneumomediastinum, and surgical emphysema. CT can confidently make the diagnosis of pneumothorax in these cases if required.

### 2.1.1.2 Aortic Dissection

Aortic dissection is a separation or splitting of the arterial wall and characteristically presents with sudden-onset, severe chest pain in the precordial and substernal region radiating through to the back. There are two types of dissection according to the Stanford anatomic classification: type A, which starts in the ascending aorta and proximal arch; and type B, which begins distal to the origin of the left subclavian artery. Type A accounts for 70% of aortic dissections and has a high incidence of complications including

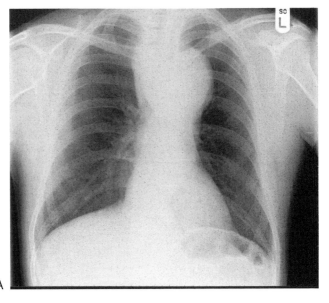

A

FIGURE 2.1.1.2A. Aortic dissection. Erect posteroanterior (PA) CXR showing widening of superior mediastinum and displacement of the trachea in a 21-year-old man after trauma.

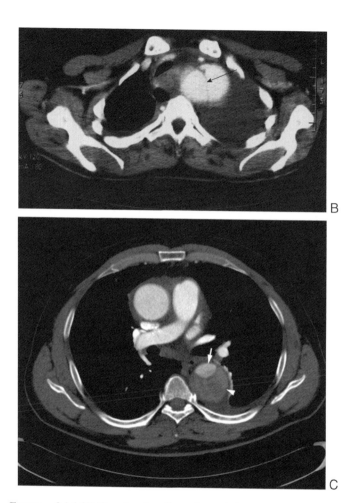

Figure 2.1.1.2B,C. Aortic dissection. (B) Contrast-enhanced CT (CECT) image showing the presence of the intimal flap (arrow) separating the true and false lumen. Note also tracheal displacement. (C) Axial CECT image of the descending aorta, the true lumen (arrow) is usually smaller and shows an earlier enhancement then the false lumen (arrowhead).

cardiac tamponade, coronary artery occlusion, acute aortic regurgitation, and dissection extension into the major aortic arch branches. Early imaging and diagnosis is essential as the treatment for type A is usually emergency surgery, whereas type B dissections have a more benign course and are managed conservatively.

Although a normal chest radiograph does not exclude the diagnosis of dissection, this should be performed initially. Suggestive signs of aortic dissection are

- Widening of the mediastinum (on an erect film taken posteroanteriorly)
- Separation of the aortic wall calcification from the margin of the aortic outline by more than 1 cm
- Depression of the left main bronchus
- Widening of the paravertebral line

If previous chest radiographs are available, comparison can be very helpful to assess any recent change in the appearance of the aortic outline and mediastinum in general.

Depending on the patients' clinical status, the availability of imaging techniques, and local expertise, different imaging routes can be followed. If the patient is relatively stable and cardiac MRI is immediately available, it is an excellent diagnostic method. MRI offers multiplanar imaging of the entire aorta with its branches as well as excellent views of the mediastinum. Subtle signs such as early intramural hematoma are particularly well demonstrated. It is usually easy to diagnose full aortic dissection with the intimal flap and the different signal intensity of blood flow in true and false lumens. The most important issue is to define the full extent of the dissection into the aortic branches as well as complications such as aortic regurgitation, which is well observed using cine sequences.

Currently, CT is more widely available than cardiac MRI, and multislice CT offers image reconstruction in different anatomic planes. It also has the advantage of showing calcification, which is of value in detecting intimal displacement. It is important to perform an unenhanced CT acquisition before administering intravenous contrast medium as acute intramural hematoma may appear as an ellipse of increased attenuation. Dynamic intravenous contrast medium–enhanced CT may show:

- Presence of the intimal flap
- Presence of the true and false lumen
- Extent of the dissection (aortic branches involved and possible infarction of intraabdominal viscera)
- Complications such as aortic rupture, pericardial collections, and so forth.

---

### Aortic Dissection

- Chest radiograph is normal in 25%.
- MRI is an excellent imaging technique where available; only for stable patients.
- CT is more widely available and is better in showing intimal calcification.
- Aortography has a limited role where CT and/or MRI are available.

---

Transthoracic and transesophageal echocardiography have a very high sensitivity and specificity in diagnosis of aortic dissection but are more operator dependent and not always available in emergency situations. Invasive aortography, formerly the routine technique for aortic dissection, is now rarely required.

### 2.1.1.3 Infections

Lower respiratory tract infection (pneumonia) may present with chest pain and is usually diagnosed with chest radiography alone. This evaluates the extent of pneumonia and its complications, assesses response to treatment, and

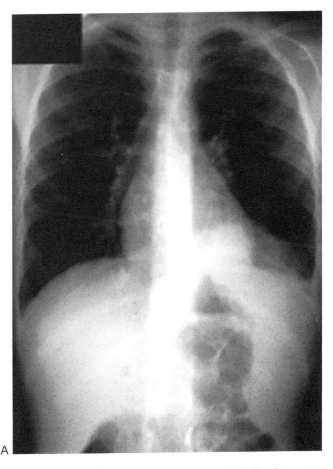

A

FIGURE 2.1.1.3A. Left lower lobe pneumonia. CXR showing a retro-cardiac opacity which is obscuring the medial aspect of the left hemidiaphragm.

FIGURE 2.1.1.3B,C. Left lower lobe pneumonia. (B) CXR showing right upper lobe pneumonia. (C) Coronal reformatted image of a CECT of the thorax in the same patient highlighting an air bronchogram (arrow).

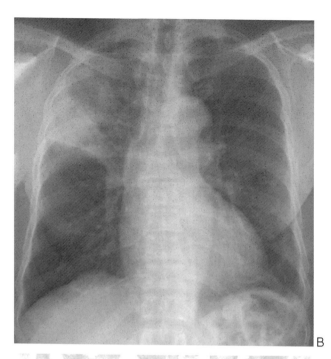

B

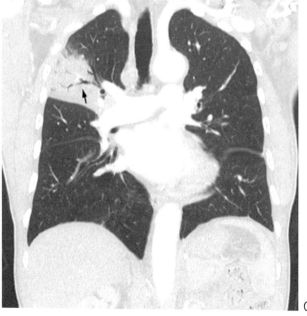

C

demonstrates possible predisposing lung pathologies. Features of pneumonia on a plain chest radiograph include:

- Area of parenchymal opacification, which may be lobar, segmental, or nonsegmental.
- Presence of an air-bronchogram.
- Localized translucencies indicating the presence of an abscess, pneumatocele formation, and so forth.
- Volume changes are not usually present unless there is associated collapse.
- Pleural effusion or empyema.
- Hydropneumothorax.
- Underlying diseases such as malignancy, bronchiectasis, pulmonary sequestration, bronchogenic cyst, and so forth, which are predisposing factors in developing pneumonia.

Comparison with previous radiographs is helpful for evaluating new changes in patients with a predisposing condition and assessing response to treatment.

## 2.1.1.4 Tumors

Chest pain may be the presenting symptom in patients with bronchial carcinoma. Pain often indicates invasion of the chest wall by the tumor and carries a poor prognosis. The diagnosis can be suggested from the plain chest radiograph, although further imaging with CT combined with bronchoscopy and biopsy is usually required for tumor staging.
Radiologic features of bronchial carcinoma include:

- Lung mass with lobular, spherical, or oval shape especially if located in the periphery, which may contain cavitation or small areas of calcification.
- Fine streaks of opacity radiating into the lung from a central mass (*corona radiata*) or a solitary band (*tail*) between the lesion and the pleura.
- Lung apex mass (superior sulcus tumor), which may resemble pleural thickening.

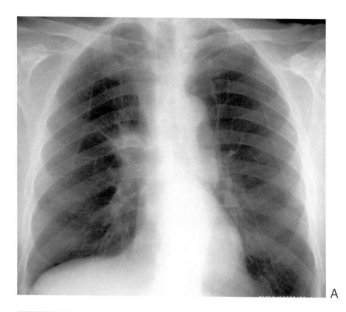

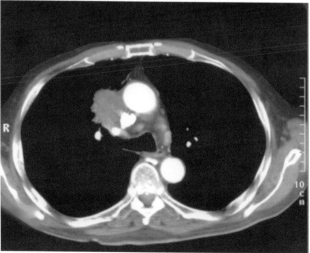

FIGURE 2.1.1.4A,B. Bronchial carcinoma. (A) CXR showing a spiculated central mass superior to the right hilum. (B) CECT showing the right central mass as well as small-volume mediastinal lymphadenopathy. (*Continued*)

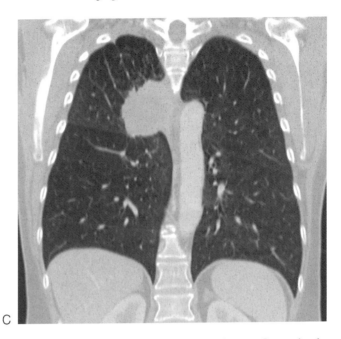

C

FIGURE 2.1.1.4C. (*Continued*) Bronchial carcinoma. Coronal reformation of this tumor using lung window setting.

- Lobar collapse in association with central tumors—adjacent fissures may show a bulge related to the proximal mass.
- The presence of consolidation in an elderly patient confined to one lobe or more that does not improve over 3 weeks despite antibiotic treatment, or recurrent consolidation in the same lobe.
- Visible mass with associated compression of major bronchi.
- Hilar enlargement/mediastinal mass.
- Pleural/pericardial effusion.
- Raised paralyzed hemidiaphragm.
- Direct chest wall invasion such as rib destruction or soft tissue mass.

# Investigation and Staging of Bronchial Carcinoma

- Plain chest radiograph and CT are the routine imaging modalities for diagnosis and intrathoracic staging.
- MRI provides additional useful information regarding involvement of great vessels, pericardium, heart, carina and aortopulmonary window and superior sulcus.
- PET provides accurate assessment of the intrathoracic lymph node involvement and is useful for evaluating recurrent disease.

CT remains superior to MRI in the diagnosis of lung lesions, especially small parenchymal lesions, near the pleura or diaphragm. PET using [$^{18}$F]fluorodeoxyglucose (FDG) has higher sensitivity and specificity than CT and MRI for diagnosing lymph node involvement by the tumor. MRI is as good as CT for the routine diagnosis of mediastinal invasion. MRI is, however, superior to CT for assessing involvement of major mediastinal blood vessels and the carina. It is better than CT in demonstrating chest wall or diaphragmatic invasion. MRI is currently the imaging modality of choice for demonstrating the extent of the superior sulcus tumor as it provides excellent tissue contrast between the tumor and the soft tissues of the chest wall, and also the thin layer of extrapleural fat is better seen on MRI than on CT.

## 2.1.1.5 Boerhaave's Syndrome

Boerhaave's syndrome is the spontaneous rupture of the distal esophagus and usually presents with acute severe chest pain. It is caused by violent retching and vomiting usually after an alcoholic binge. The sudden increase in the intraluminal pressure causes a full-thickness esophageal tear. It is

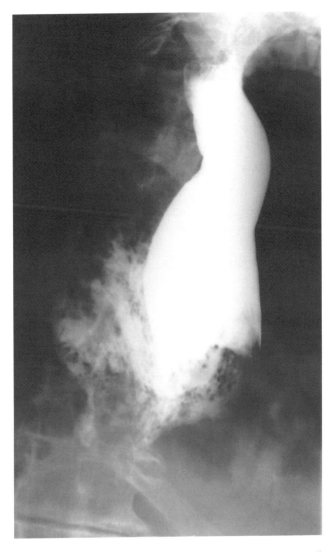

FIGURE 2.1.1.5. Boerhaave's syndrome. Water-soluble swallow showing extravasation of the contrast medium from the distal esophagus into the mediastinum.

the most serious perforation of the GI tract carrying a very high mortality rate (70%). The tear is vertical and typically measures 1 to 4 cm. It is most commonly located on the left lateral wall of the distal esophagus, just above the gastroesophageal junction. Rarely, it occurs in the cervical or upper thoracic esophagus where it has a better prognosis.

Prompt imaging is crucial, as large tears often require immediate surgical intervention. Plain chest radiograph findings include:

- Widening of the mediastinum
- Pneumomediastinum: manifest by radiolucent air streaks along the lateral border of aortic arch and descending thoracic aorta
- Left-sided pleural effusion

CT in the imaging test of choice but is usually unable to locate the exact anatomic site of esophageal tear. CT demonstrates:

- Extraluminal air
- Extravasation of oral contrast medium in the lower mediastinum surrounding the esophagus
- Pleural and/or pericardial fluid collections

X-ray swallow with water-soluble contrast media shows extravasation from the distal esophagus into the mediastinum and extension into the adjacent fascial planes with large tears.

## Suggestions for Further Reading

1. Greene R, McCloud TC, Stark P. Pneumothorax. Semin Roentgenol 1977;12:313–325.
2. Khan IA, Nair CK. Clinical, diagnostic, and management perspectives of aortic dissection. Chest 2002;122(1):311–328.
3. Set PAK, Flower CDR, Smith IE, et al. Hemoptysis: comparative study of the role of CT and fiberoptic bronchoscopy. Radiology 1993;189:677–680.
4. Laurent F, Montaudon M, Corneloup O. CT and MRI of lung cancer. Respiration 2006;73(2):133–142.
5. Nehoda H, Houmont K. Boerhaave's syndrome. N Engl J Med 2001;344:138–139.

## 2.1.2 Abdominal Pain

Patients with acute abdominal pain present a diagnostic and management challenge to the general surgeon. Plain abdominal radiographs remain the first imaging investigation in these patients and may provide a specific diagnosis in some cases. Increasingly, additional imaging with US, CT, and MRI is performed early in the management of these patients to facilitate a rapid definitive diagnosis.

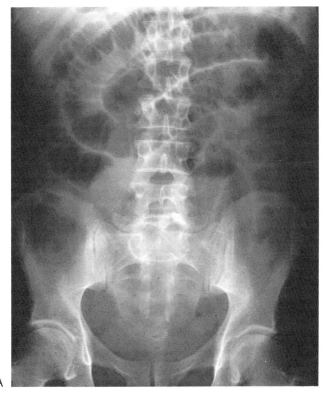

A

FIGURE 2.1.2A. Small bowel obstruction. Supine abdominal X-ray (AXR) showing multiple dilated gas-filled loops of small bowel.

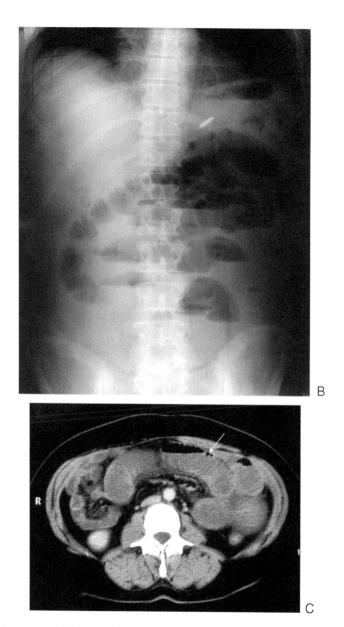

FIGURE 2.1.2B,C. Small bowel obstruction. (B) Erect AXR on the same patient showing multiple fluid levels. (C) CECT (different patient) showing dilated loops of small bowel with the *string of beads* sign (arrow). (*Continued*)

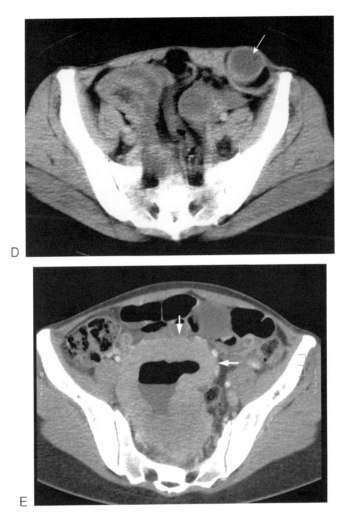

Figure 2.1.2D,E. (*Continued*) Small bowel obstruction. (D) CECT on the same patient showing a Spigelian hernia (arrow) as the cause of the small bowel obstruction. (E) Axial CECT showing extensive wall thickening of the ileum causing small bowl obstruction Histology revealed a primary small bowl lymphoma.

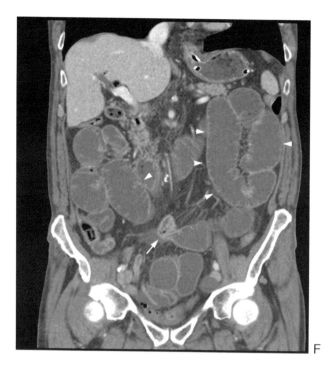

F

FIGURE 2.1.2F. Small bowel obstruction. Coronal reformatted images of CECT of a different patient with small bowel obstruction due to adhesions; note the transition zone (arrow) and the dilated bowel loops (arrowheads).

## 2.1.2.1 Small Bowel Obstruction

In mechanical small bowel obstruction (SBO), swallowed air and intestinal secretions fill the dilated proximal small bowel and there is reduction in the caliber and gas content of large bowel distal to the obstruction. Features of SBO on plain abdominal radiograph are

- Dilated gas-filled loops of small bowel, greater than 3-cm diameter, which tend to be central, numerous, and in the case of the jejunum have valvulae conniventes that extend right across the bowel.

- Multiple fluid levels on an erect abdominal radiograph.
- *String of beads* sign on an erect abdominal radiograph, due to small amount of gas trapped between valvulae conniventes.
- The small bowel may be completely filled with fluid, especially with a longer standing degree of obstruction, giving the appearance of "gasless" abdomen.
- Absence of gas or feces in the large bowel.
- All the above signs may be absent in proximal SBO, where a dilated stomach may be the only sign.

These changes may appear after 3 to 5 hours and are usually present after 12 hours from the onset of symptoms. Often, the plain abdominal radiograph will not show the cause of obstruction, but there are several important causes that should be diagnosed on plain radiographs. The presence of gas below the line of the inguinal ligament may indicate an incarcerated femoral or inguinal hernia, a cause of SBO in about 15% of cases. Gas in the biliary tree and an opaque gallstone in the right iliac fossa are the classic features of a gallstone ileus. It should be remembered that adhesive disease is the cause of SBO in about 50% of cases.

CT will confirm the presence of SBO and also provide additional information regarding the level and the cause of obstruction. It will, in addition, give staging information if a malignancy is the cause of SBO. CT is the imaging technique of choice in diagnosis of small bowel strangulation, being of great value in urgent surgical management of these patients.

## 2.1.2.2 Large Bowel Obstruction

The most common cause of large bowel obstruction (LBO) in the Western world is a tumor, with rectosigmoid carcinoma being the most common (65% at this location). This is closely followed by diverticulitis. Because LBO affects much more commonly the left colon, plain abdominal radiographs usually suggest the diagnosis. Dilated (more than 5-cm diameter), gas-filled loops of large bowel that tend to be peripheral and few in number are seen proximal to the level

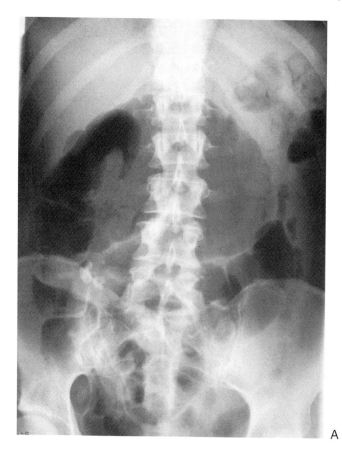

A

FIGURE 2.1.2.2A. Cecal volvulus. Supine AXR showing a large gas-filled viscus in the center of the abdomen. (*Continued*)

of obstruction with little or no gas present distal to it. If the ileocecal valve is competent, little or no gas is seen in the small bowel, whereas multiple dilated gas-filled small bowel loops are present when the ileocecal valve is incompetent. In the latter, the appearances can be identical with pseudoobstruction (see later). With long-standing obstruction, the cecum is at risk of perforation.

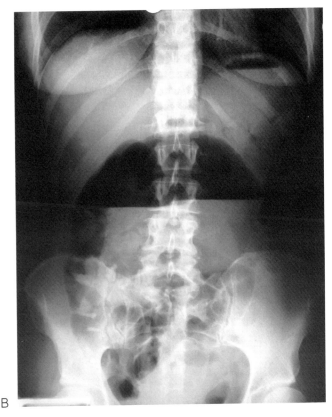

B

FIGURE 2.1.2.2B. (*Continued*) Cecal volvulus. Erect AXR showing an air-fluid level within the dilated cecum.

Single-contrast enema is often performed as an emergency investigation prior to surgery in order to confirm the presence and determine the level of obstruction. Usually, the information provided by the combination of plain abdominal radiograph and contrast enema is adequate for appropriate surgical management. In the situations when the plain radiograph findings are equivocal or when the patient is unable to tolerate a contrast enema, CT can provide comparable infor-

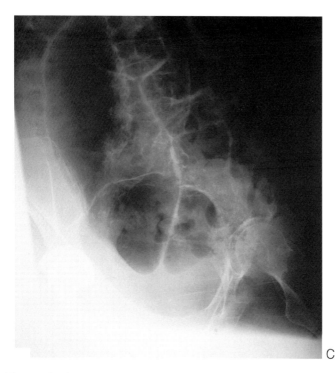

C

FIGURE 2.1.2.2C. Cecal volvulus. Sigmoid volvulus. Supine AXR showing a markedly dilated loop of sigmoid colon with a distinct midline crease that corresponds with twisted mesenteric root (*coffee bean* sign).

mation regarding the level and cause of obstruction as well as staging information if a colonic carcinoma is demonstrated.

*Cecal volvulus* is a surgical emergency, and the diagnosis can be promptly made on a plain abdominal radiograph with no need for further imaging. Features of cecal volvulus are

- Markedly dilated cecum containing few haustral markings.
- Large gas-filled viscus, which may lie virtually anywhere in the abdomen but is more frequently positioned in the left upper quadrant.

- Marked gaseous or fluid distension of the small bowel, which also fills the empty right iliac fossa.
- Attached gas-filled appendix.
- Collapse of the left side of the colon.

*Sigmoid volvulus* usually occurs in the elderly or in institutionalized psychiatric patients. The diagnosis should be confidently made on a plain abdominal radiograph. Barium enema may be used in equivocal cases. Features of sigmoid volvulus are

- A dilated ahaustral bowel loop with apex under the left hemidiaphragm, above the level of the T10 vertebra.
- *Coffee bean* sign: markedly dilated loop of sigmoid colon with a distinct midline crease that corresponds with twisted mesenteric root.
- *Bird of prey* sign: tapered end of barium column on barium enema.

### 2.1.2.3 Pseudoobstruction

Pseudoobstruction, or Ogilvie's syndrome, is marked colonic distension without a mechanical obstructing cause that may occur as a result of pharmacological, biochemical, neural, endocrine, and myopathic factors. It usually occurs in the elderly patient and may be self-limiting or associated with common medical conditions such as chest infection, myocardial infarction, and so forth. Plain abdominal radiographs may be indistinguishable from LBO, demonstrating dilated large and small bowel loops, and a single-contrast enema or CT is usually indicated to exclude mechanical obstruction in order to avoid inappropriate surgical intervention, which can be disastrous.

### 2.1.2.4 Perforation of Hollow Viscus

The most common cause of pneumoperitoneum is perforation of peptic ulcer followed by diverticulitis and malignancy. An erect chest radiograph and an abdominal radiograph, usually taken supine, should always be obtained

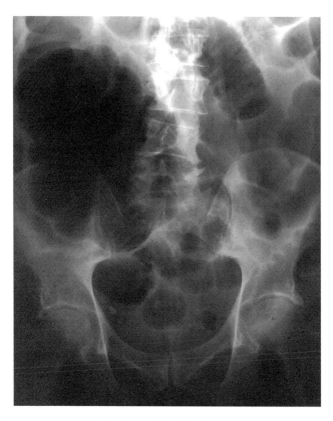

FIGURE 2.1.2.3. Pseudoobstruction. Supine AXR showing dilated large and small bowel loops. Note the enormous distension of the cecum.

if perforation is suspected. Both are very sensitive, and as little as 1 mL of free air can be detected on an erect chest radiograph or a left lateral decubitus abdominal radiograph. On the erect chest radiograph, air is seen under one or both diaphragms and if under both results in the *continuous diaphragm* sign.

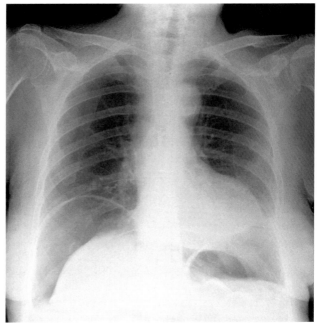

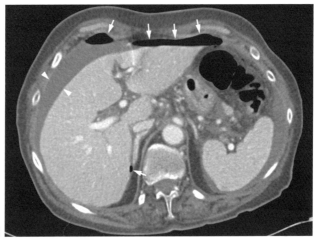

FIGURE 2.1.2.4A,B. Perforation of hollow viscus. (A) Erect CXR showing large amount of free subdiaphragmatic air. (B) CECT demonstrating free intraperitoneal air (arrows) and fluid (arrowheads) after gastric perforation.

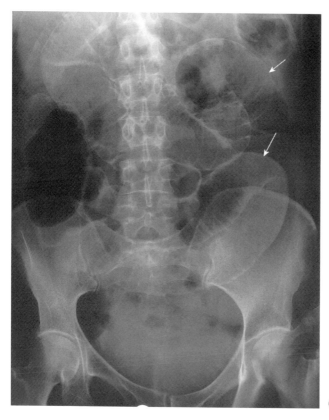

C

FIGURE 2.1.2.4C. Perforation of hollow viscus. Supine AXR in the same patient showing *Rigler's* sign (arrows).

Signs of free intraperitoneal air on a supine abdominal radiograph are

- Air overlying or outlining solid organs such as liver and spleen (*lucent liver* sign)
- A triangle of air outlining Morrison's pouch (*Doges cap* sign)
- Air outlining intraabdominal structures such as falciform ligament, umbilical median, medial and lateral ligaments (*inverted V* sign)

- Bowel wall outlined by air both inside and outside (*Rigler's* sign)
- Centrally placed intraperitoneal free air (*football* sign) and scrotal air in children
- *Cupola* sign of air under the central diaphragm

It is very important to be able to recognize conditions that can simulate pneumoperitoneum because an observational error may lead to unnecessary surgery. Chilaiditi's syndrome in which the colon is interposed between the liver and the diaphragm can mimic pneumoperitoneum, but usually haustral folds can be seen that will allow identification of the colon. A gas-containing subphrenic abscess may also mimic a pneumoperitoneum as can basal pulmonary atelectasis. On the left side, a gas-distended fundus of the stomach may cause confusion, and clarification by a decubitus film may be necessary. Postoperative air may sometimes cause confusion, but this should have resolved by 5 to 7 days and should decrease in size with time.

Where the plain radiographs are equivocal, then CT is the most sensitive imaging technique for diagnosis of free intraperitoneal air. A small amount of free intraabdominal air can be seen anterior to the liver or midline abdomen (as the mobile air collects anteriorly with the patient in the supine position) and in the peritoneal recesses or retroperitoneal spaces. This is best appreciated by reviewing the images on "lung window" settings. CT may identify the cause of pneumoperitoneum and can offer additional information to plain radiographs. X-ray contrast studies can also be performed to confirm a perforation. Water-soluble contrast medium administered orally or via a nasogastric tube combined with fluoroscopic imaging can often identify the location of a perforation in the proximal GI tract. Urgent surgery is usually required for a perforated hollow viscus.

## 2.1.2.5 Acute Appendicitis

Acute appendicitis is the most common cause of an abdominal surgical emergency. The diagnosis is usually made on the basis of clinical history and physical examination with no need for imaging. Sometimes, however, the clinical findings are equivocal, and increasingly CT is used to confirm the diagnosis, although concerns about radiation exposure indicate that it should only be used when appropriate.

## Plain Abdominal Radiograph Findings in Acute Appendicitis

- Calcified appendicolith (10%)
- Right iliac fossa mass
- Localized ileus
- Loss or right psoas margin and blurring of properitoneal fat line
- Extraluminal gas collections
- Pneumoperitoneum
- Scoliosis concave to the right

Plain abdominal radiographic findings are nonspecific and usually unhelpful. They may show an appendicolith. CT is the most accurate technique for confirming the diagnosis of appendicitis and assessing the severity and possible complications, with a sensitivity and specificity of 100% and 95%, respectively. CT findings include a distended appendix measuring more than 6 mm in diameter, which is thick-walled and may enhance after administration of intravenous contrast medium. An appendicolith can be seen in 25% of the cases. Associated inflammatory changes include streaking of the periappendiceal fat, fluid collection owing to abscess formation, thickening of the cecal and/or terminal ileum wall, and thickening of the anterior renal and adjacent fascial planes.

Graded-compression US has a recognized value in the diagnosis of acute appendicitis in children. Graded

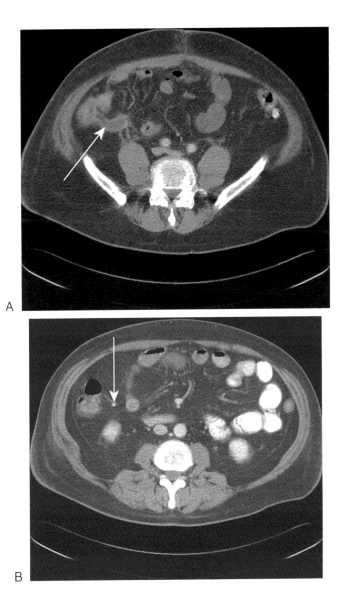

A

B

FIGURE 2.1.2.5A,B. Acute appendicitis. (A) CECT demonstrating a dilated appendix (arrow). Note the enhancement of the wall of the appendix and stranding of the pericecal fat planes. (B) An appendicolith (arrow) is noted.

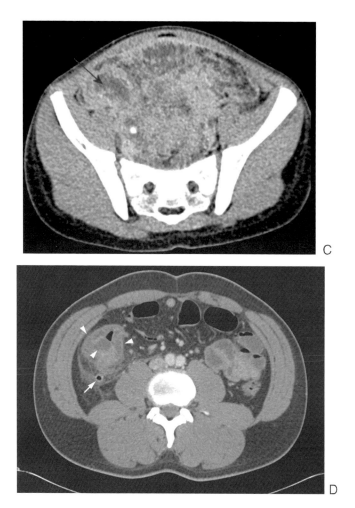

FIGURE 2.1.2.5C,D. Acute appendicitis. (C) CECT axial. (D) CECT in a different patient with appendicitis (arrow) and abscess formation in the wall of the cecum (arrowheads). Note that it is unusual to see the presence of luminal area in acute appendicitis. (*Continued*)

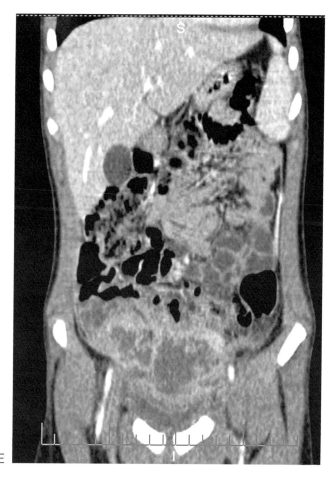

E

FIGURE 2.1.2.5E. (*Continued*) Acute appendicitis. Coronal reformatted images (different patient) demonstrating an appendicular
abscess (arrow). An appendicolith is again noted.

compression is applied with the transducer over the right
iliac fossa in order to displace bowel gas and examine
the appendix. In a patient with appendicitis, the appendix
appears as a tubular noncompressive, aperistaltic structure
that measures more than 7 mm in its transverse diameter. An

appendicolith, casting posterior acoustic shadowing, may be seen. The surrounding inflammatory mass appears heterogeneous, and an abscess or fluid collection may be present. US in expert hands potentially offers a sensitivity and sensitivity of 98%. The choice between US and CT depends on the local availability and expertise, but US is preferred in children and pregnant women because of lack of ionizing radiation and in younger women where there is higher incidence of pelvic inflammatory disease. Imaging, however, should not be a substitute for adequate clinical skills and should only be requested when there is clinical uncertainty, thus avoiding the delay in prompt surgical treatment or inappropriate radiation exposure.

### 2.1.2.6 Acute Cholecystitis

Acute cholecystitis results from cystic duct obstruction by an impacted gallstone in more than 90% of cases. Patients usually present with classic symptoms and signs of right upper quadrant pain and tenderness, and the diagnosis will be confirmed by US if surgery is contemplated during the first admission. Apart from confirming the diagnosis, US may detect other causes of acute abdominal pain such as right renal obstruction.

## Ultrasound Features in Acute Cholecystitis

- Gallstone: mobile hyperechoic foci that cast posterior acoustic shadowing
- Tenderness on compression over the gallbladder (sonographic *Murphy's* sign)
- Thickening of gallbladder wall greater than 3 mm
- Pericholecystic fluid
- Distended gallbladder

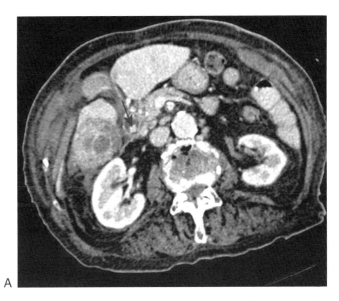

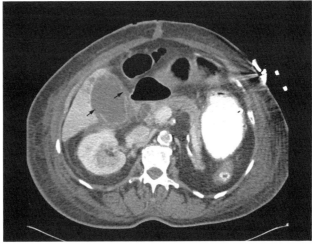

FIGURE 2.1.2.6A,B. Acute cholecystitis. (A) CECT showing an inflamed gallbladder and a calcified stone in the common bile duct (arrow). (B) Axial CECT in a septic patient showing lack of mucosal enhancement of the gallbladder (arrows) suggestive of a necrotizing cholecystitis.

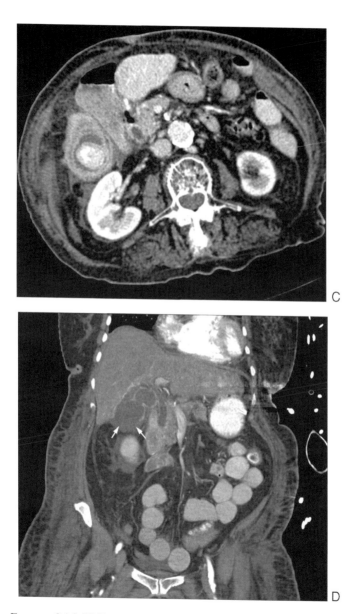

FIGURE 2.1.2.6C,D. Acute cholecystitis. (C) Note the dilated gallbladder with enhancing, thickened wall and stranding of the surrounding fat planes as well as the large laminated gallstone. (D) Coronal reformatted image of this CECT showing the extent of the necrosis (arrows).

Plain abdominal radiograph findings are nonspecific and usually unhelpful. They include calcified gallstones (20%), right upper quadrant mass due to an enlarged gallbladder, duodenal or high colonic ileus, and rarely air within the biliary tree (in cases of gallstone ileus).

On US, the two most important features are the presence of gallstones and maximal tenderness on compression over the gallbladder (sonographic *Murphy's* sign), which is highly specific for acute cholecystitis. Both scintigraphy using technetium-99m ($^{99m}$Tc)-labeled derivatives of iminodiacetic acid (HIDA) and US are diagnostically accurate, and the choice between them may reflect local expertise and availability. HIDA scintigraphy has a 100% negative predictive value and a good sensitivity. A positive examination consists of nonvisualization of gallbladder but prompt visualization of the common bile duct and duodenum 1 hour after injection. False-positive results occur in alcoholic liver disease and in patients receiving parenteral nutrition.

CT is not the primary imaging modality because of its low sensitivity for gallstones. It is, however, of good value in imaging possible complications such as gangrenous cholecystitis, perforation of gallbladder resulting in abscess formation or biloma, Mirizzi's syndrome, and so forth.

## 2.1.2.7 Acute Pancreatitis

The most common cause of acute pancreatitis in Western countries is alcohol followed by cholelithiasis. Less frequent causes are metabolic disorders such as hyperparathyroidism, trauma, abdominal surgery, viral infections, drugs, and so forth. The plain abdominal radiograph is unreliable, being normal in more than 75% of patients with acute pancreatitis, but can demonstrate a number of features (see box).

---

# Plain Film Findings in Acute Pancreatitis

- Gallstones
- Pancreatic calcifications with chronic pancreatitis
- Gasless abdomen
- Generalized or paralytic ileus in the left upper quadrant
- Sentinel loop and colon cutoff sign
- Separation of greater curve of stomach from transverse colon
- Loss of left psoas outline
- Extraluminal air bubbles
- Left pleural effusion
- Elevated left hemidiaphragm

---

The diagnosis of acute pancreatitis is usually straightforward based on clinical history, findings, and hyperamylasemia. In these cases, US is primarily indicated to detect the presence of gallstones as a possible cause because the pancreas is not always visible due to the accompanying small bowel ileus. When visualized, the pancreas may be enlarged, hypoechoic, and ill defined. Peripancreatic fluid and possible complications such as abscess and pseudocyst formation can be identified. US is unable to accurately assess pancreatic necrosis, which many consider the single most important determinant of morbidity and mortality in these patients.

CT more reliably demonstrates all these features (except for gallstones). In particular, it is the imaging technique of choice to assess the presence and extent of pancreatic necrosis. After intravenous contrast medium administration, thin, small field of view sections are obtained during pancreatic phase enhancement in addition to conventional arterial and venous phases. In cases of mild acute pancreatitis, the pancreas may appear normal. More commonly,

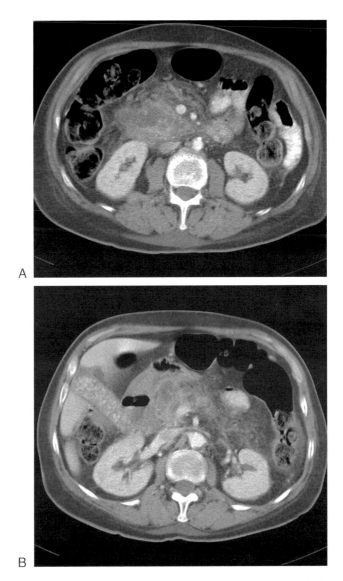

FIGURE 2.1.2.7A,B. Acute pancreatitis. (A) CECT showing inflammatory changes mainly involving pancreatic head, which appears enlarged and contains areas of lack of parenchymal enhancement suggestive of edema. (B) There are numerous gallstones within the gallbladder.

the gland appears enlarged with increased attenuation in the peripancreatic fat and adjacent fascial plane thickening. The pancreas itself normally shows homogeneous enhancement, but in severe acute pancreatitis necrotic tissue appears as areas of reduced or absent enhancement in the parenchyma. The presence of parenchymal air is highly suggestive of infection although fistulation to the gastrointestinal tract can result in identical appearances. CT is very sensitive for demonstrating complications such as pancreatic abscess, adjacent fluid collections, or pseudocyst formation. It is particularly helpful for vascular complications including both pseudoaneurysm formation and thrombosis of the splenic or portal vein. The Balthazar CT Severity Index, which has been shown to have a good correlation with morbidity and mortality of the disease, can be calculated on the basis of the CT findings.

---

## Recommendations for Contrast-Enhanced CT in Acute Pancreatitis

- Patients who do not improve within 72 hours of the commencement of conservative management
- To confirm the diagnosis of acute pancreatitis and to evaluate the extent and severity of disease
- Patients with a Ranson score greater than 3
- To diagnose complications
- To guide interventional procedures

---

### 2.1.2.8 Small Bowel Ischemia

Different processes can lead to small bowel ischemia, the most common being mesenteric thrombus or embolus, infiltration, and trauma. It represents a serious surgical condition that can be difficult to diagnose clinically and often requires prompt imaging and treatment.

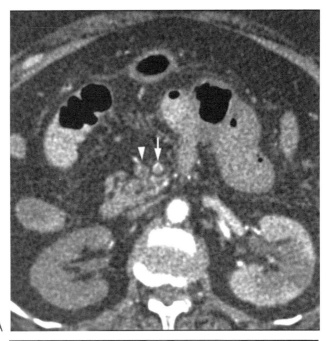

A

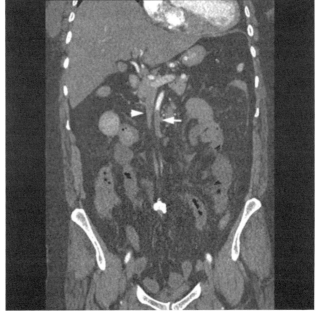

B

FIGURE 2.1.2.8A,B. Small bowel ischemia. (A) Axial and (B) coronal reformatted images of a CECT study showing filling defects within the superior mesenteric artery (arrow) and vein (arrowhead).

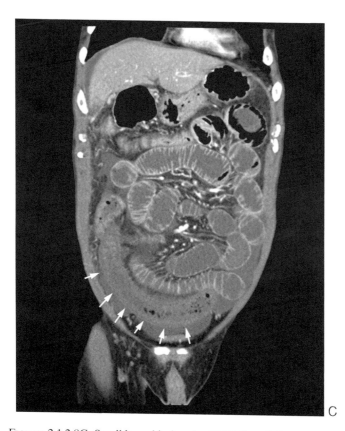

C

FIGURE 2.1.2.8C. Small bowel ischemia. CECT in a different patient demonstrating an abnormal loop of small bowel that shows a thickened and unenhancing wall (arrows).

Plain abdominal radiographic findings depend on the severity of the disease. Nonspecific dilated bowel loops with multiple fluid levels or fluid-filled loops are a frequent finding. Thickening of the bowel wall ("thumb printing") may be visible, which is due to submucosal hemorrhage and edema. In severe cases, gas may be seen within the bowel wall and/or the mesenteric and portal veins. Barium studies will show separation of the bowel loops and thickening of valvulae conniventes. Mucosal ulceration can be seen in advanced cases.

Contrast-enhanced CT may provide an early diagnosis of mesenteric ischemia by demonstrating not only the dilated fluid-filled loops of bowel with wall thickening and ascites but more importantly the lack of mesenteric vascular enhancement after administration of intravenous contrast media. Occasionally, thrombus may be visible in a mesenteric artery or vein and gas within the mesenteric veins and/or bowel wall. Reconstruction of vascular anatomy using multislice CT will further assist in an accurate diagnosis.

Angiography was widely used to make the diagnosis prior to CT and remains valuable for equivocal cases. It will show features of occlusion, vasoconstriction, or vascular beading. Emboli are typically seen at major branching points distal to the first 3 cm of superior mesenteric artery.

## 2.1.2.9 Renal Colic

Renal colic is usually caused by stone disease but may also arise secondary to a transitional cell carcinoma of the renal pelvis or ureter. Microscopic or macroscopic hematuria occurs in most cases.

FIGURE 2.1.2.9A,B. Urolithiasis. (A) Axial CT image showing a left distal ureteric stone. (B) CT coronal reformatted image confirming the presence of the left distal ureteric stone approximately 5 cm from the left vesico-ureteric junction. Also note mild dilatation of the left ureter proximal to the stone. (*Continued*)

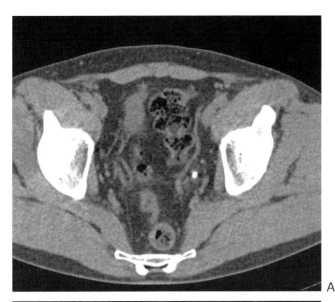

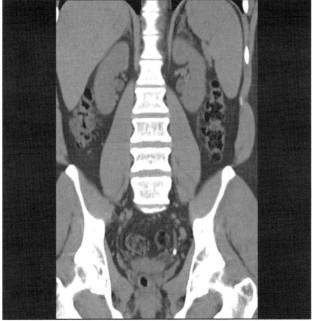

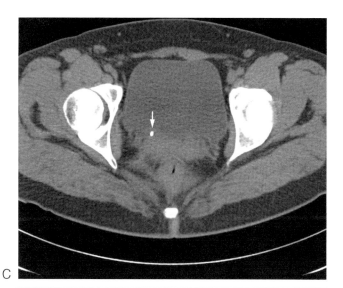

C

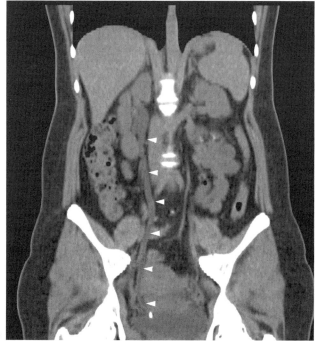

D

FIGURE 2.1.2.9C,D. (*Continued*) Urolithiasis. (C) Axial CECT of an impacted right vesico-ureteric junction (VUJ) calculus (arrow). (D) Curved planar reformatted image of the right dilated ureter (arrowheads).

*Urolithiasis:* Imaging is almost always required to make an initial diagnosis but may not be needed for uncomplicated recurrent disease. Plain abdominal radiograph may show a calcified opacity along the line of the urinary tract, but up to 30% of the stones are not calcified (or obscured). Intravenous urography (IVU) is helpful in showing the degree and site of obstruction. Features of obstruction include dilatation of the pelvicaliceal system and/or the ureter, depending on the position of the stone. US may show renal stones and features of hydronephrosis, but it has to be remembered that the pelvicaliceal system may appear normal in the early phase of obstruction. US cannot reliably demonstrate ureteric stones. Nonenhanced CT (NECT) is increasingly used as the imaging modality of choice when urolithiasis is suspected. It has a sensitivity and specificity of 97%, with a calculus within the ureter being pathognomonic. It can detect radiolucent stones as well as ureteric edema surrounding a small impacted stone. Stranding of the perinephric/periureteral fat and perinephric fluid collections are associated findings easily detectable by CT. Confusion can arise from the presence of phleboliths, but multiplanar reformats in coronal and sagittal planes will help resolve the dilemma.

*Transitional cell carcinoma:* Plain abdominal radiograph is usually normal. IVU shows single or multiple filling defects in the renal pelvis, ureter, or bladder. One or more calyces may also fail to opacify (*phantom calyx*) or there may be calyceal distension with tumor (*oncocalyx*). Hydronephrosis due to tumor obstruction is an additional but uncommon finding. US confirms these findings, but CT is indicated for staging purposes.

## 2.1.3 Abdominal Sepsis

Patients with abdominal sepsis may present with local or systemic signs and frequently pose a diagnostic and management challenge to the surgeon. Imaging is important for both diagnosis and therapy, as image-guided drainage of intraabdominal collections is often the preferred treatment option. This section concentrates on imaging of abdominal collections and the postoperative abdomen.

### 2.1.3.1 Intraabdominal Collections

Patients with abdominal sepsis may present with fever; abdominal pain, and/or bowel symptoms caused by subphrenic, intrahepatic, and pelvic abscesses.

*Subphrenic and subhepatic* abscesses can occur after surgery of stomach, pancreas, spleen, splenic flexure of colon, perforating cholecystitis, or gastric and duodenal ulcer or can develop as a complication of acute pancreatitis, appendicitis, cholecystitis, and perforated duodenal ulcer. A *right paracolic* abscess can follow acute appendicitis or develop secondary to a subphrenic abscess, whereas a *left paracolic* abscess can result from perforated diverticular disease or from ascending pelvic infections. A pelvic abscess may complicate appendicitis, pelvic inflammatory disease, and large bowel surgery. Abscesses also occur within organs such as liver, pancreas, and spleen.

A plain chest radiograph may show a raised hemidiaphragm, loculated gas under the diaphragm, or basal lung consolidation and/or pleural effusion. The abdominal radiograph can demonstrate gas fluid level or gas bubbles that remain unchanged on sequential films. Other features include a soft tissue mass, paralytic ileus, or effacement of the fat planes.

US is an appropriate technique for suspected collections in the upper abdomen and pelvis if localizing signs are present but may overlook collections. This is a particular problem in the iliac fossae due to overlying bowel gas. Collections appear as hypoechoic or anechoic lesions usually with irregular margins and may be multiloculated. CT is the modality of choice for studying the whole abdomen and pelvis. Fluid collections are well demonstrated, and rim enhancement around

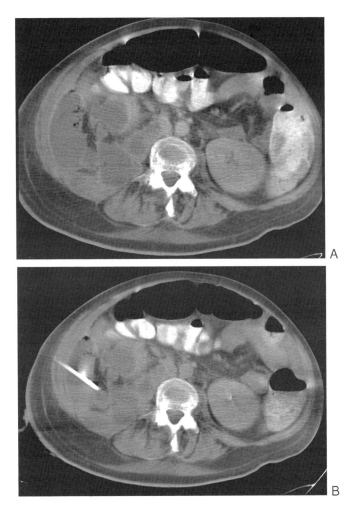

FIGURE 2.1.3.1A,B. Right paracolic abscess. (A) CECT showing a large multiloculated collection in the right paracolic space. Note the presence of rim enhancement. (B) CT-guided insertion of drain into the abscess.

a collection after contrast media injection strongly suggests an abscess. Good bowel preparation by oral contrast media is essential to distinguish fluid-filled bowel loops from an abnormal collection. Both US and CT can guide percutaneous aspiration and drainage. MRI is not widely used for acute intraabdominal sepsis but is particularly helpful in preoperative imaging of pelvic fistulae due to inflammatory bowel disease, most commonly Crohn's disease.

In the majority of the patients, the diagnosis is established by CT and/or US, but when those are negative or when there are no localizing signs of the sepsis, a labeled white cell scintigram is a useful diagnostic option. It offers a sensitivity and specificity of 95% and 90%, respectively. Acute intraabdominal sepsis can be investigated using either indium-111 ($^{111}$In) or $^{99m}$Tc-labeled white cells, although the latter gives images of better resolution and is preferred if there is coexistent inflammatory bowel disease. Sequential imaging is essential in order not to miss an abscess in communication with bowel lumen.

---

## Imaging of Abdominal Sepsis

- US is a good initial imaging method for upper abdomen and pelvis when localizing signs are present, but *not* for the iliac fossae where obscuring gas may lead to false-negative results.
- CT is the modality of choice for diagnosis where localizing signs to the upper abdomen or true pelvis are absent.
- Both US and CT can be used for guiding percutaneous aspiration and drainage where appropriate.
- White cell scanning is an alternative investigation when there are no localizing signs. It demonstrates enteric communication and can identify sepsis at any site.
- MRI is very helpful is cases of inflammatory bowel disease complicated by perineal fistulae.

---

In patients with genuine pyrexia of unknown origin, gallium-67 ($^{67}$G) should be the first imaging option. This is because only 10% of cases with pyrexia of unknown origin (PUO) are caused by pyogenic sepsis, and in the absence of neutrophils, a labeled white cell scintigram will not be positive. Other conditions such as lymphoma, melanoma, tuberculosis, sarcoidosis, and so forth, show avid gallium uptake, making it nonspecific in imaging of the abdominal sepsis. The value of gallium imaging is to localize a potential cause that can subsequently be investigated by other imaging modalities such as US, CT, or MRI.

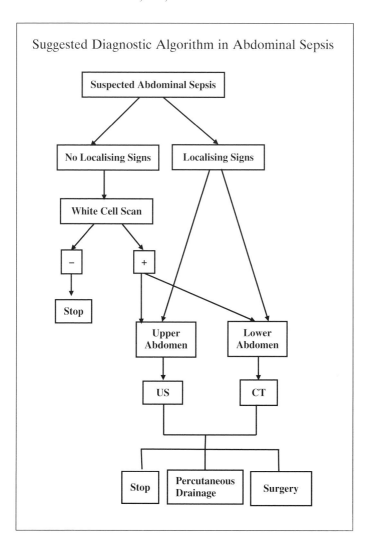

Suggested Diagnostic Algorithm in Abdominal Sepsis

## 2.1.3.2 Imaging of Postoperative Abdomen

Imaging is valuable for investigating postoperative complications. The clinical picture may be that of an acute abdomen or intraabdominal sepsis. Plain abdominal radiographs still remain the first imaging test, and the same diagnostic criteria as for the preoperative radiograph apply. As mentioned before, both US and CT are used to detect abnormal fluid collections, abscesses, and so forth, but CT is usually the more practical option because it provides a rapid, noninvasive, and global view of the abdominal cavity, unimpeded by extensive bowel gas from concomitant ileus, wounds, surgical dressings, and so forth.

Pneumoperitoneum is a common feature on the postoperative plain abdominal radiograph, being present in 60% of postlaparotomy patients. Intraperitoneal air takes between 1 day and 3 weeks to reabsorb dependent on the patient's body habitus. Gas is more rapidly reabsorbed in obese patients who generally have no residual gas after the fifth postoperative day. It is important to note that any increase in the amount of postoperative air indicates an anastomotic leak or a hollow viscus perforation. CT is the most sensitive method for the assessment of pneumoperitoneum and will also detect abnormal air collections in abdominal viscera.

Paralytic ileus is common and may simulate or coexist with obstruction. Small bowel obstruction due to adhesions may develop a few days after a laparotomy. Patients may develop anastomotic leaks and/or intraabdominal abscesses. Imaging features of these conditions are described in detail in the previous sections.

## Suggestions for Further Reading

1. Marincek B. Nontraumatic abdominal emergencies: acute abdominal pain: diagnostic strategies. Eur Radiol 2002;12(9): 2136–2150.
2. Stapakis JC, Thickman D. Diagnosis of pneumoperitoneum: abdominal CT versus upright chest film. J Comput Assist Tomogr 1992;16:713–716.

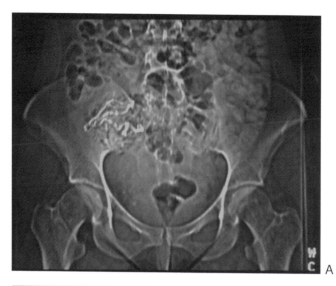

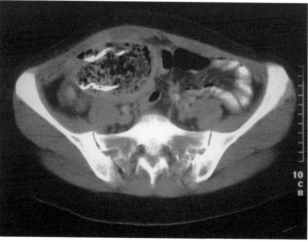

FIGURE 2.1.3.2A,B. Imaging of postoperative abdomen. (A) Scanogram and (B) axial CECT images showing a retained swab as demonstrated by the radiopaque material. Note extensive mass due to gossypiboma.

3. Rao PM, Boland GWL. Imaging of acute right lower abdominal quadrant pain. Clin Radiol 1998;53:639–649.
4. Ng CS, Watson CJ, Palmer CR, et al. Evaluation of early abdominopelvic computed tomography in patients with acute abdominal pain of unknown cause: prospective randomised study. BMJ 2002;325:1387–1390.
5. Lee R, Tung HKS, Tung PHM, et al. CT in the acute mesenteric ischaemia. Clin Radiol 2003;58:279–287.

# 2.2 Mass

## 2.2.1 Imaging of Abdominal Masses by Their Location

Many intraabdominal tumors when advanced may present as palpable abdominal masses. Imaging confirms and diagnoses these masses and is particularly helpful for diagnosing and detecting smaller tumor masses that are not easily palpable.

This section concentrates on imaging of tumors of liver, adrenal, body and tail of pancreas, retroperitoneal lymphadenopathy, and sarcomas. Imaging of pancreatic head tumors is described under "Jaundice" (Section 2.4) imaging features of renal cell carcinoma are given in under "Hematuria" (Section 2.3.2), and imaging of gastrointestinal tumor is described in detail under "Bleeding" (Section 2.3).

### 2.2.1.1 Liver Tumors

Liver tumors can be classified as primary and metastatic tumors. Primary tumors may be benign or malignant. US is widely used in liver imaging, especially for the follow-up of the patients with cirrhosis, to detect small hepatocellular carcinomas. Other benign lesions, such as hemangiomas, adenomas, or focal nodular hyperplasia (FNH), can be detected incidentally during US. Capillary hemangiomas are the most common benign tumors of the liver and have a classic appearance on US examination of a well-defined hyperechoic, often slightly lobulated mass. Unfortunately, this appearance may be mimicked by some metastases, particularly from the gastrointestinal tract, so in the appropriate clinical situation further imaging may be required. US findings on focal nodular hyperplasia and adenoma are usually nonspecific. MRI is now considered the most sensitive and specific imaging technique for the diagnosis of these benign liver lesions. Hemangiomas are of high signal intensity, similar to water and higher than spleen, on T2-weighted (T2W) images. They rapidly enhance in a centripetal fashion after gadolinium diethylenetriamine penta-acetic acid (Gd-DTPA) administration (*light bulb* sign.) FNH appears as an isointense to minimally hypointense lesion on T1-weighted (T1W) images and hyperintense on T2W images. The central scar, if present, is of low signal intensity on T1W images and of high signal intensity on T2W images. After Gd-DTPA injection, the lesion enhances avidly and homogeneously while the central scar remains initially of low signal intensity, although it may demonstrate delayed enhancement. On MRI examination, simple adenoma has similar appearances to FNH.

Combination of US and triphasic contrast-enhanced CT (CECT) can accurately suggest a definitive diagnosis in most cases of malignant liver lesions. This section provides a detailed description of imaging findings in hepatocellular carcinoma and liver metastasis.

*Hepatocellular carcinoma* (HCC) is the most common primary liver tumor. It may present either as a single large mass or as a multifocal diffuse lesion. The tumor usually develops in a cirrhotic liver, for example, due to chronic viral hepatitis (HBV and HCV cirrhosis) but can occur de novo within a normal liver. In cirrhotic livers, all imaging techniques have limited sensitivity and specificity. US is widely used as a screening technique for at-risk patient groups and may demonstrate a hypoechoic, heterogeneous, and less frequently a hyperechoic lesion. Features of underlying liver cirrhosis such as a small, nodular hyperechoic liver with associated splenomegaly, varices, and ascites can be well appreciated on US.

HCC appears as a low-attenuation single or multifocal mass on unenhanced CT images and necrosis, calcification,

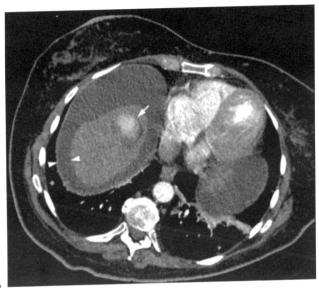

A

FIGURE 2.2.1.1A. Hepatocellular carcinoma. Arterial phase of a CECT demonstrating an enhancing lesion in the superior aspect of the right lobe of the liver (arrow) consistent with hepatocellular carcinoma. Note the presence of ascites (arrowheads).

and fat may be demonstrated. Biphasic CECT, with arterial and portal phase imaging, increases the sensitivity of the technique as approximately 10% of HCC lesions are only visible during the arterial phase. The tumor shows heterogeneous enhancement on arterial phase images and appears as a heterogeneous low-attenuation lesion, sometimes indistinguishable from normal liver parenchyma, on portal phase images. HCC demonstrates intense enhancement on CT hepatic arteriography. There is no enhancement during CT arterial portography.

FIGURE 2.2.1.1B,C. Liver metastasis. Portal phase (B) axial and (C) coronal CECT images demonstrating multiple low-attenuation lesions within both lobes of the liver consistent with multiple liver metastasis.

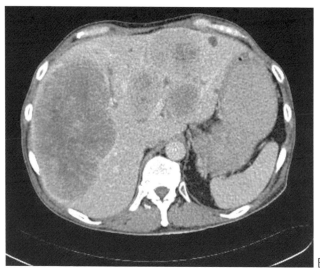

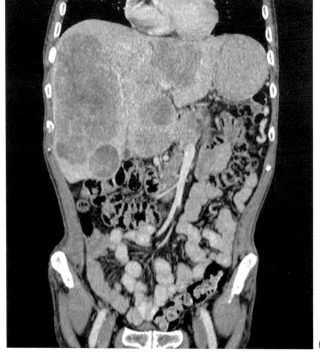

Frequently, it can be very difficult to distinguish HCC from regenerating cirrhotic nodules on US and CT images. MRI can be helpful in these cases. HCC appears hypointense on T1W images and hyperintense on T2W images, and cirrhotic nodules may demonstrate increased signal intensity on T1W images and low signal intensity on T2W images. The use of liver-specific contrast medium agents, such as super paramagnetic iron oxide (SPIO), may improve the sensitivity of MRI in detecting small HCC. Magnetic resonance angiography (MRA) allows noninvasive, accurate assessment of hepatic vessels, portal vein, and inferior vena cava prior to hepatic resection or liver transplantation.

Angiography typically demonstrates a hypervascular tumor with marked neovascularity and arteriovenous shunting.

*Liver metastases* may be demonstrated with US, CT, or MRI with an increasing order of sensitivity. Although they have relatively specific features, they may be mimicked by benign causes such as liver abscesses, hemangiomas, and so forth. A tissue diagnosis is therefore appropriate, and where impossible (such as lesions less than 5 mm), serial follow-up imaging is indicated.

US typically demonstrates multiple solid liver lesions with a hypoechoic rim. Biopsy of larger lesions can be performed under US guidance and is especially useful when the liver is the only site of metastasis and the primary tumor is unknown. CT is excellent in demonstrating liver metastasis especially when larger than 10 mm. They can be hypovascular such as those from lung, gastrointestinal tract, pancreatic, bladder, uterine tumors, most breast cancer cancers, and so forth, or hypervascular in cases of renal cell carcinoma (RCC), thyroid carcinoma, melanoma, endocrine tumors, and so forth. Although the majority of lesions are detectable on unenhanced CT, the addition of CECT (portal phase images) increases the sensitivity by 5% to 10%. Typically, CT demonstrates randomly distributed lesions throughout the liver with low-attenuation center and peripheral rim enhancement in case of hypovascular metastasis. Hypervascular metastases appear as high-attenuation lesions in late arterial phase images. MRI is also a comparably accurate technique for demonstrating liver metastasis but is not routinely used in practice owing to availability and costs compared with US or CECT examinations. [$^{18}$F]fluorodeoxyglucose–positron emission tomography (FDG-PET) is increasingly used where hepatic resection of a solitary metastasis is being considered, but mainly for the detection of extrahepatic metastatic disease.

## 2.2.1.2 Adrenal Tumors

The detection of adrenal masses has significantly increased with the widespread use of cross-sectional imaging, and they are revealed in 5% to 10% of CT or magnetic resonance (MR) examinations of the abdomen. The majority of adrenal masses are incidental benign adenomas, even in patients with known primary malignancy. However, the adrenal is a common site of metastasis, particularly from lung, breast cancer, and melanoma primaries. The accurate differentiation between an adenoma and a metastasis becomes crucial in patients with known primary malignancy, particularly lung cancer, as adrenal metastasis indicates advanced disease and curative surgery is not warranted. In practice, a combination of CT, MRI, and PET is used to characterize adrenal masses in the oncology patient.

Certain CT findings such as the shape of the gland, size of the lesion, and change in size over time are useful in differentiating benign from malignant lesions. Adenomas tend to have smooth margins, are smaller, and show little change over time. Large lesions (especially if greater than 3 cm) that increase in size with time and have an irregular contour are likely to represent adrenal carcinomas or metastasis. These features are useful but nonspecific. There are two main criteria used to reliably differentiate benign adenomas from malignant lesions: intracellular lipid content and vascular enhancement pattern. A dedicated adrenal CT protocol should be performed. It consists of an NECT followed by a CECT with images obtained in portal (70 seconds)

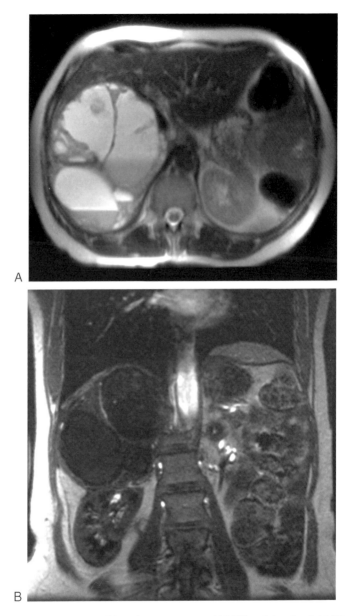

FIGURE 2.2.1.2A,B. Pheochromocytoma. (A) T2-weighted axial MR showing a large, high signal intensity mass in the right adrenal. (B) The mass is of low signal intensity on T1-weighted coronal image. Appearances are in keeping with an adrenal pheochromocytoma.

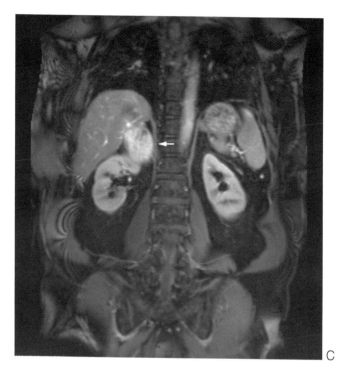

C

FIGURE 2.2.1.2C. Pheochromocytoma. Typical contrast enhancement (arrow) on a coronal T1-weighted, fat-suppressed sequence of a right adrenal pheochromocytoma (different patient).

and delayed phases (10 to 15 minutes). Thin collimation (3 mm) and rapid bolus injection of intravenous contrast medium (3 mL/s) are used. The majority of adenomas (80%) contain intracellular lipid that results on low attenuation <10 Hounsfield units (HU) on NECT, thus reliably distinguishing them from malignant lesions, and no further imaging is required. Around 20% of adenomas are lipid-poor making differentiation from malignant lesions practically impossible on NECT alone. The attenuation value and percentage enhancement washout of the lesion at delayed CECT are very useful in these cases. A HU of less than 37 on delayed images and 50% or greater enhancement washout value is diagnostic of an adenoma (sensitivity of 96% and specificity of 100%).

It is important to realize that if CT findings are still equivocal, the patient should undergo further evaluation with MRI or an adrenal biopsy to confirm a benign or a malignant lesion. Conventional T1W, T2W, and Gd-DTPA enhanced images and chemical shift imaging are used. Adenomas are of low signal, whereas metastases are of high signal intensity on T2W images. However, there is significant overlap between the two. Enhancement pattern is similar to that seen during CT imaging. Chemical shift or in-phase and out-of-phase imaging is used to detect lipid and relies on the different resonance frequency rates of protons in fat and water molecules. It is the most sensitive method for differentiating adenomas from metastasis. Adenomas appear darker on out-of-phase than on in-phase images as a result of signal reduction due to cancellation of the lipid and water proton signals. In adrenal metastases, which do not contain lipid, there is no signal loss on out-of-phase images, and thus the relative signal intensity remains the same on both sequences. More recently, PET has been used in the evaluation of the nonfunctioning adrenal masses. Unlike previously discussed imaging modalities, a positive PET study accurately identifies a malignant mass rather than an adenoma. As with other tumors, PET is not reliable in diagnosis of small lesions (less than 10 mm).

Adrenal carcinomas are rare, presenting as large, usually unilateral adrenal masses. The patient may present with a palpable mass, abdominal pain or, in 50% of cases, the Cushing syndrome. The CT appearance is that of a large mass (>5 cm) with central necrosis and calcifications (20%) that shows heterogeneous contrast medium enhancement. Tumor extension into the renal vein and inferior vena cava (IVC) can be reliably identified on CT. MRI is especially helpful in evaluating IVC invasion and delineating tumor-liver interface in right adrenal carcinomas.

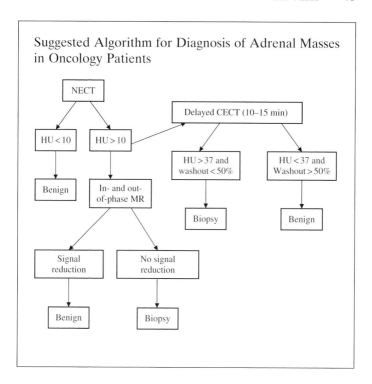

Suggested Algorithm for Diagnosis of Adrenal Masses in Oncology Patients

### 2.2.1.3 Tumors of the Pancreas

Pancreatic tumors may arise from the endocrine or exocrine pancreatic tissue. Ductal adenocarcinoma is the most common pancreatic tumor arising from the ductal epithelium of the exocrine pancreas. They occur in the pancreatic head in 65% of cases, with the remainder arising in the body or tail. Imaging features of ductal carcinoma of the pancreatic head are discussed in Section 2.4.1.3.

US is commonly the first imaging test performed to investigate jaundice or nonspecific abdominal pain. A tumor has lower reflectivity than pancreatic tissue, and obstruction of the main pancreatic duct (normally <3 mm diameter) may also be apparent. CECT with thin collimation (3 mm) and rapid intravenous bolus contrast medium injection is the technique of

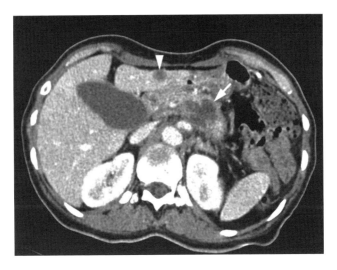

FIGURE 2.2.1.3. Carcinoma of the body of the pancreas. CECT image demonstrating a low-attenuation mass (arrow) within the normal enhancing pancreatic body representing a pancreatic duct carcinoma. Note the presence of a single metastases within the left lobe of the liver (arrowhead).

choice for both diagnosis and staging of the disease. Images are taken at different phases of contrast enhancement (i.e., arterial and portal phases). The tumor is seen as a low-attenuation area within the densely enhancing normal pancreatic tissue, better appreciated in the arterial phase. CT is capable of demonstrating perivascular invasion of arterial and venous structures such as the superior mesenteric artery, superior mesenteric vein, and splenic vein. This is crucial in the determination of tumor resectability. Complete circumferential vascular encasement by tumor is a sign of nonresectability. CT is also very sensitive in detecting invasion of other adjacent structures as well as regional lymphadenopathy and liver metastasis. Fine-needle aspiration cytology and biopsy samples can be obtained under CT guidance. Further imaging may be obtained by endoscopic or laparoscopic US. Although MRI may be helpful to evaluate vascular invasion, generally it offers no diagnostic improvement compared with CT and is not therefore routinely indicated.

## 2.2.1.4 Retroperitoneal Sarcoma

Retroperitoneal sarcoma is a primary malignant retroperitoneal tumor of mesodermal origin. It is usually a large heterogeneous mass that displaces the retroperitoneal

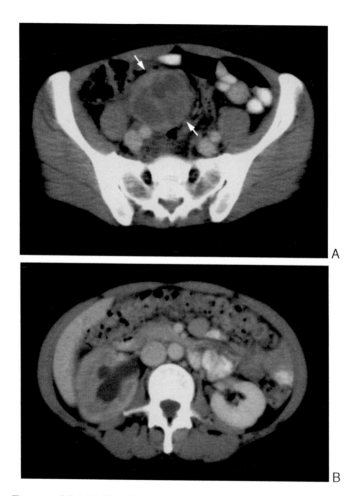

A

B

FIGURE 2.2.1.4A,B. Retroperitoneal sarcoma. CECT images demonstrating a pelvic mass (arrows in A) of mixed attenuation that is causing right-side hydronephrosis (B). Histology showed a retroperitoneal liposarcoma.

structures. Based on the tissue of origin, retroperitoneal sarcoma comprises a spectrum of malignant tumors such as liposarcoma, leiomyosarcoma, fibrosarcoma, rhabdomyosarcoma, angiosarcoma, and so forth. Liposarcoma is the most common primary retroperitoneal malignant tumor and is classically located in the perinephric region.

CT is the best imaging modality for diagnosis and staging of liposarcomas. It shows a poorly defined or well-encapsulated large mass that can be of soft tissue, fatty, or mixed attenuation depending on histologic differentiation. The mass may contain areas of calcifications and can invade, displace, or distort surrounding structures. It usually shows heterogeneous enhancement on CECT. MRI demonstrates variable signal intensity that depends on the amount of fat content as well as intratumoral necroses and hemorrhage. Liposarcomas are hypovascular on angiography.

## 2.2.2 Abdominal Aortic Aneurysm

The plain abdominal radiograph is unreliable in the diagnosis of abdominal aortic aneurysm (AAA) and any suspected rupture. Positive signs when present (approximately 70%) depend on the outlining of an aneurysm by wall calcification or perhaps a retroperitoneal mass. US is very useful in diagnosis and defining aneurysm diameter (the most important determinant of rupture risk) but may be limited with regard to relationship with renal arteries and aortic bifurcation. However, if the aneurysm commences below the level of the superior mesenteric artery, it is unlikely that the renal arteries are involved. US can also show the presence of thrombus and detect free intraabdominal fluid in a leaking AAA. It is widely used to follow aneurysm growth when resection is deferred.

CT is the investigation of choice in patients who are being considered for aneurysm resection. It provides an accurate measurement of aneurysm diameter and wall thickness and is useful in evaluating the degree of aortic calcification and presence of thrombus. Classification of AAA into suprarenal,

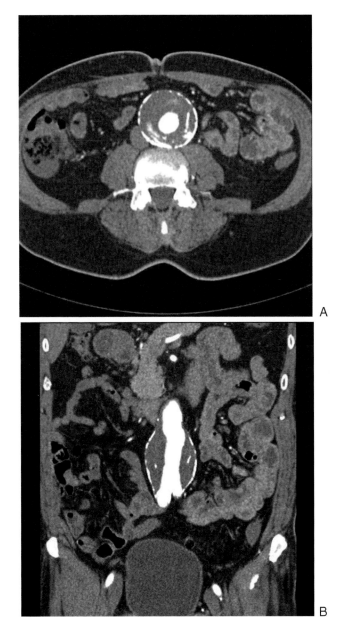

FIGURE 2.2.2A,B. Abdominal aortic aneurysm. CT angiogram (A) axial, (B) coronal. (*Continued*)

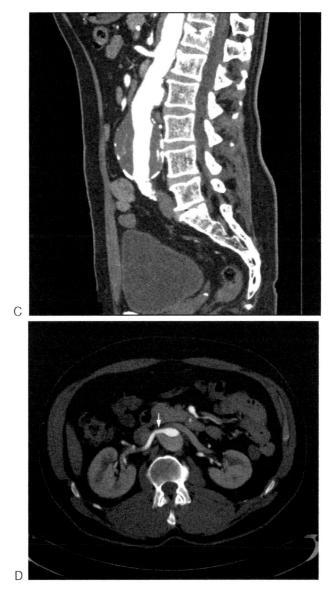

FIGURE 2.2.2C,D. (*Continued*) Abdominal aortic aneurysm. CT angiogram (C) sagittal images showing an aortic abdominal aneurysm. (D) Axial CECT image of an abdominal aortic aneurysm with dissection. Note the origin of the right renal artery (arrow) from the true lumen.

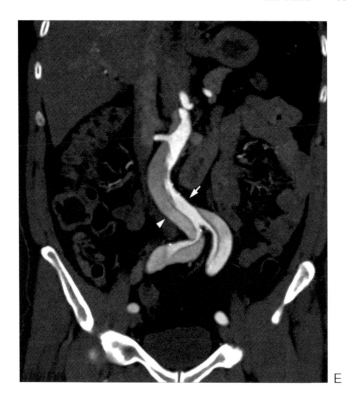

E

FIGURE 2.2.2E. Abdominal aortic aneurysm. Coronal reformatted image of the same patient, showing the extent of the dissection; the true lumen (arrow) is significantly smaller than the false lumen (arrowhead).

pararenal, and infrarenal is fundamental to the surgical approach and is easily achieved with CT angiography using multislice CT and three-dimensional reconstruction. CT also routinely demonstrates anatomic variants such as retroaortic left renal vein, left-sided inferior vena cava, horseshoe kidney along with complications such as leakage, inflammatory aneurysms, and periaortitis. Postoperatively, CT evaluates leakage, abscess formation, and complications such as aorto-duodenal fistula, and so forth.

MRI, especially MRA, equals CT for vascular assessment preoperatively but is not widely used owing to relative cost and availability. X-ray–based angiography is now rarely required prior to surgery as multislice CT and MRI usually provide adequate information.

## Suggestions for Further Reading

1. Kamel IR, Choti MA, Horton KM, et al. Surgically staged focal liver lesions: accuracy and reproducibility of dual-phase helical CT for detection and characterisation. Radiology 2003;227: 752–757.
2. Caoili EM, Korobkin M, Francis IR, et al. Adrenal masses: characterisation with combined unenhanced and delayed enhanced CT. Radiology 2002;222:629.
3. Mehmet Erturk S, Ichikawa T, Sou H, et al. Pancreatic adeno-carcinoma: MDCT versus MRI in the detection and assessment of locoregional extension. J Comput Assist Tomogr 2006;30(4): 583–590.
4. Kim T, Murakami T, Oi H, et al. CT and MR imaging of abdominal liposarcoma. AJR 1996;166:829–833.
5. Iino M, Kuribayashi S, Imakita S, et al. Sensitivity and specificity of CT in the diagnosis of inflammatory abdominal aortic aneurysms. J Comput Assist Tomogr 2002;26:1006–1012.

## 2.3 Bleeding

Both gastrointestinal hemorrhage and hematuria are common clinical problems and may require significant imaging investigations.

## 2.3.1 Gastrointestinal Bleeding

Gastrointestinal (GI) hemorrhage can be anatomically divided into upper GI bleeding, defined as hemorrhage from a site proximal to the ligament of Treitz, whereas bleeding distal to this point is lower GI in origin. Diagnostic techniques include endoscopy, angiography, and nuclear medicine.

## 2.3.1.1 Diagnosis of Upper Gastrointestinal Bleeding

Endoscopy is the primary technique for diagnosis and therapeutic intervention in upper GI hemorrhage (e.g., esophageal varices).

*2.3.1.1.1 Endoscopy*  Whenever GI bleeding is thought to originate from a site proximal to the ligament of Treitz, the principal investigation technique should be flexible upper GI endoscopy. The diagnostic accuracy is excellent if it is performed within the first 12 hours of bleeding. Endoscopy is widely available and relatively noninvasive. It is of great value as it can qualitatively assess the bleeding rate and the possibility of rebleeding and allows biopsies to be obtained. It provides a definitive diagnosis in the majority of the cases

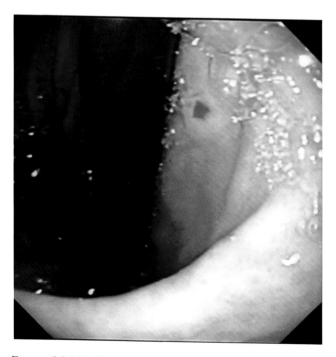

FIGURE 2.3.1.1.1. Endoscopy. Dieulafoy lesion in the stomach.

and offers numerous therapeutic interventions for specific lesions (i.e., injection of adrenaline into the base of the ulcer or hot biopsy of small bleeding sources). If the bleeding lesion is still thought to be high small bowel (i.e., around or distal to the ligament of Treitz), then upper GI enteroscopy is indicated.

*2.3.1.1.2 Angiography* Angiography is only performed when full endoscopy fails to locate a bleeding point or when therapeutic embolization is indicated. Selective injection of celiac axis and superior mesenteric artery is performed. In cases of active blood loss (bleeding rate >0.5 mL/min), extravasated contrast medium is seen into the bowel lumen. Angiography is insensitive if bleeding is intermittent or of venous origin. Angiography is valuable in detection of vascular abnormalities such as arteriovenous malformations and angiodysplasia.

*2.3.1.1.3 Nuclear Medicine Studies* Nuclear medicine studies, either $^{99m}$Tc-labeled red cells or sulfur colloid, are rarely used in the diagnosis of upper GI hemorrhage. A bleeding point shows as an area of increased uptake outside normal areas of uptake. Radionuclide studies are more sensitive than angiography but lack accuracy in localizing the site of bleeding.

## 2.3.1.2 Causes of Upper Gastrointestinal Bleeding

There are numerous causes of upper GI bleeding, most of them now amenable to medical rather than surgical treatment. They are listed in the following subsections.

*2.3.1.2.1 Esophagitis, Ulcers, and Varices* Esophagitis commonly results from gastroesophageal reflux disease (GORD), which is a manifestation of peptic ulcer disease. GORD causes a spectrum of abnormalities ranging from superficial esophagitis to deep penetrating ulcers. It accounts for approximately 3% of upper GI bleeding. Barrett's esophagus also results from GORD, wherein the normal squamous epithelium of the distal esophagus is replaced by

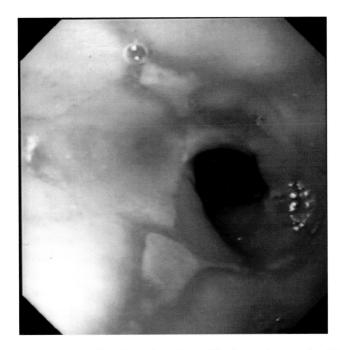

FIGURE 2.3.1.2.1. Esophageal erosions. Classic erosive esophagitis with the presence of reflux ulcers in the lower esophagus.

specialized columnar epithelium. Ulcers when they occur in this situation are found at the squamo-columnar junction. Barrett's esophagus is associated with a high incidence of adenocarcinoma so that patients with this condition are kept under surveillance with yearly endoscopy and biopsy to detect early dysplastic changes.

Esophageal varices can be demonstrated either by endoscopy or barium studies. Endoscopy is advantageous as it also offers the therapeutic options of injecting sclerosants or banding the varices. There are two types of varices: uphill and downhill varices. Uphill varices are seen in portal hypertension and are caused by the diverted blood flow via the esophagus to the superior vena cava. They are found in the lower esophagus and fundus of the stomach. Downhill varices are caused by superior vena cava obstruction, where the blood flow is diverted from head and neck via esophagus to the azygos system. They are usually found in upper and mid esophagus. At barium swallow, both types appear as serpiginous filling defects best seen in prone position.

*2.3.1.2.2 Gastric Erosions and Peptic Ulceration*    Gastro-duodenal erosions account for the majority of gastrointestinal hemorrhages. Gastric erosions are aphthous ulcers that do not penetrate the muscularis mucosa. Alcohol, salicylates, and nonsteroidal anti-inflammatory drugs (NSAIDs) are the most common causes of acute hemorrhagic gastritis. Another important cause is the stress syndrome in critically ill patients due to multiple trauma, sepsis, shock, and so forth.

At double-contrast barium studies, gastric erosions appear as shallow, small, 1- to 2-mm-diameter collections of barium surrounded by a radiolucent rim of edema; an appearance mirrored at endoscopy with a hemorrhagic center and edematous rim.

The majority of peptic ulcers in the stomach or duodenum are related to *Helicobacter pylori* infection and the remainder due to NSAID and alcohol abuse. Most gastric ulcers are benign. They are usually situated on the lesser curve and on the posterior wall of the antrum and body of the stomach. Ulcers occurring on the fundus and the proximal half of the greater curve are more likely to be malignant. Gastric ulcers related to NSAIDs and alcohol are more commonly seen on the greater curve of the antrum. Gastric ulcers at any location can cause major hemorrhage due to the high vascularity of the stomach wall, typically via the left gastric artery. Duodenal ulcers are virtually always benign and are 3

FIGURE 2.3.1.2.2A,B. Gastric erosions. (A) Classic erosive antral gastritis most likely associated with NSAID use. (B) Small discrete ulcers with evidence of recent bleeding (different patient). The arrow indicates the pylorus.

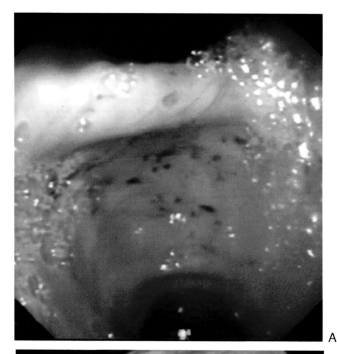

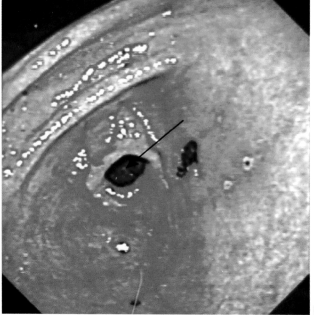

times more frequent than gastric ulcers. The majority (95%) of duodenal ulcers occur in the duodenal bulb, 5% being postbulbar. The latter may raise the possibility of Zollinger-Ellison syndrome. Most bleeding duodenal ulcers are situated in the posterior wall of the duodenal bulb, where they erode the gastroduodenal artery.

The majority of the peptic ulcers are diagnosed by endoscopy but do exhibit classic appearances on double-contrast barium studies. The appearance depends on whether the ulcer is seen in profile or en face. In profile, the classic feature of a benign ulcer is the sign of penetration (i.e., the ulcer crater projects through the wall of the stomach). It may demonstrate a thin lucent line representing intact mucosa (Hampton line) or edema around the margin may cause the so-called ulcer collar. Sometimes, the edema may be so prominent that it results in an ulcer mound that projects into the lumen of the stomach. Seen en face, the ulcer is demonstrated as a collection of barium with folds radiating to it, and these usually fade gently as they reach the edge of the ulcer. Likewise, duodenal ulcers may be seen as an ulcer crater but also cause deformity of the duodenal cap, particularly when associated with scarring from healing fibrosis (*Trefoil deformity*).

CT is not a sensitive imaging tool for diagnosis of simple peptic ulcer disease, but it is very useful in the diagnosis of complications such as ulcer penetration or perforation. Imaging features include thickening of the stomach/duodenal wall, luminal narrowing, and infiltration of surrounding fat or organs such as pancreas. CT is the best test for diagnosis of free air in the abdomen (duodenal and antral ulcers) or in the lesser sac (ulcers of the posterior body of the stomach).

*2.3.1.2.3 Tumors of the Upper Gastrointestinal Tract*    Gross bleeding is unusual from tumors of esophagus, stomach, or small bowel, but occult upper GI hemorrhage resulting in anemia is common. Significant bleeding occasionally complicates gastric tumors, particularly ulcerated gastrointestinal stromal tumors (GISTs).

Gastrointestinal stromal tumor is a submucosal mesenchymal tumor that originates from smooth muscle cells. It can occur anywhere in the GI tract, the stomach being the most common site. At barium studies, it appears as a rounded, exophytic submucosal mass that can ulcerate. Contrast-enhanced CT demonstrates a hypervascular submucosal mass on arterial phase images and helps demonstrate the common exophytic element. Necrosis is a common feature of large lesions. On MRI, it appears as an isointense mass on T1W sequences and hypointense to isointense with hyperintense areas of necrosis on T2W sequences. They enhance after gadolinium administration.

Gastric carcinoma is the third most common GI malignancy. Diagnosis by double-contrast barium meal has been largely replaced by endoscopy, which also offers simultaneous biopsy. Staging is performed by endoscopic US (local) and CT (distant).

At double-contrast barium meal, early gastric cancer appears as either an elevated polypoid lesion, or a superficial plaque-like lesion, or as a shallow irregular ulcer. Advanced gastric cancer has different appearances in barium studies. It may be ulcerative, polypoid, or infiltrative. A malignant ulcer has irregular borders with lobulated folds converging toward the crater when viewed en face. In profile, the ulcer often has an intraluminal location and demonstrates an abrupt acute angle at its margin with normal mucosa. Polypoid cancer shows as a smooth or lobulated filling defect, whereas the infiltrative variety narrows the lumen and when extensive results in a linitis plastica appearance (5% to 15%).

CT offers good delineation of the primary tumor if water is used as intraluminal contrast agent. CT findings include a polypoid mass with or without ulceration, focal or diffuse thickening of stomach wall with loss of normal rugae, and stranding of perigastric fat. Mucinous carcinoma demonstrates areas of low attenuation and calcifications within the thickened gastric wall. Scirrhous carcinoma produces thickened gastric wall that shows marked enhancement on dynamic CT study.

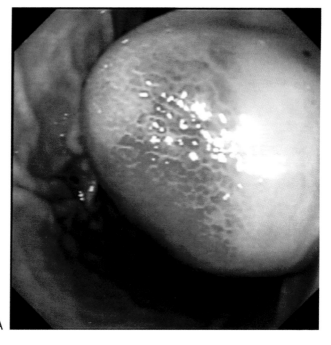

A

FIGURE 2.3.1.2.3A. Gastrointestinal stromal tumor. Large, smooth submucosal mass with evidence of early mucosal ulceration.

⟶

FIGURE 2.3.1.2.3B,C. Gastrointestinal stromal tumor. Axial CECT images of an extensive peritoneal bleeding originating from tumor erosion (not shown) of jejunal artery. Note the contrast agent extravasation (arrow in B) indicating the origin of the bleeding.

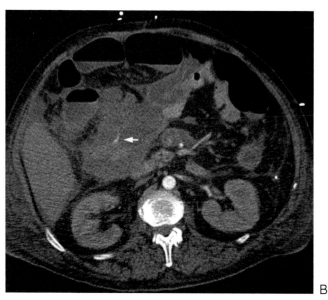

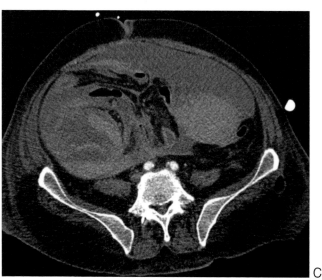

## 2.3.1.3 Diagnosis of Lower Gastrointestinal Bleeding

The selection of appropriate diagnostic and therapeutic strategies is dependent on the severity and nature of the lower GI hemorrhage. These include urgent nuclear medicine study, angiography, and colonoscopy.

*2.3.1.3.1 Nuclear Medicine Studies* Nuclear medicine studies have excellent sensitivity (more than 90%) in detecting continued acute bleeding in hemodynamically stable patients. They can detect bleeding as low as 0.1 mL/min. In addition, nuclear scintigraphy is a very useful screening test prior to angiography, allowing specific angiographic approach to the appropriate mesenteric vessel. The disadvantage includes low specificity especially for small bowel lesions and lack of any therapeutic options causing possible delays in patient's management.

Technetium sulfur colloid is sensitive in detecting active bleeding, but significant hepatic and splenic uptake may obscure bleeding sites in the upper abdomen. $^{99m}$Tc-labeled red cell imaging is relatively time consuming but allows repeated imaging for up to 24 hours after injection, which is very important in cases of intermittent bleeding. It also provides better anatomic localization compared with sulfur colloid. Red cell scintigraphy has a very high negative predictive value (more than 90%) (i.e., a negative red cell study indicates that the patient has stopped bleeding). A positive test indicates continuing bleeding, and once the anatomic site of bleeding is determined, either angiographic or surgical control can be attempted.

*2.3.1.3.2 Angiography* Angiography can detect bleeding with rates as low as 0.5 mL/min. This technique requires selective catheterization of mesenteric vessels and injection of contrast medium. Extravasation and pooling of contrast medium into the bowel lumen indicates active bleeding. Direct catheterization of the appropriate vessel can be performed if bleeding site has been localized by nuclear medicine studies. The superior mesenteric artery is catheterized and injected initially, and if this fails to demonstrate bleeding, then the inferior mesenteric artery and, if necessary, the celiac trunk are studied next. Angiography offers the possibility of therapeutic options such as intraarterial infusion of vasopressin or transcatheter embolization using coils or Gelfoam (Pfizer Manufacturing, Pharmacia & Upjohn Company, Belgium).

*2.3.1.3.3 Colonoscopy*   The role of emergency colonoscopy in patients with major ongoing lower GI hemorrhage remains controversial. Technical difficulties in these cases include impaired visualization by active bleeding or blood clots and inability to identify anatomic sites within the colon. Furthermore, the risk of colonic perforation is higher in the emergency situation when compared with elective colonoscopy. Colonoscopy is very useful in cases of self-limited major hemorrhage when both nuclear medicine and angiographic studies have failed to diagnose bleeding. It also provides useful information regarding the etiology of bleeding and allows a variety of therapeutic modalities such as electrocauterization, sclerotherapy, laser photocoagulation, and so forth.

*2.3.1.3.4 Capsule Endoscopy*   In this procedure, the patient swallows a small capsule that is capable of transmitting images to an external receiver. This is proven to be particularly useful in demonstrating causes of obscure small bowel bleeding but must be used with caution if there is a possibility of a small bowel stricture.

## 2.3.1.4 Causes of Lower Gastrointestinal Bleeding

*2.3.1.4.1 Diverticular Disease*   Diverticular disease is the most common colonic pathology in Western society and is found in more than 50% of individuals over the age of 60 years. Diverticula can occur anywhere in the colon but are most common in the sigmoid colon. They represent acquired herniation of mucosa and submucosa through the muscularis propria layer of the bowel wall. Most of them are therefore false diverticula, containing only mucosa and submucosa. They usually measure 5 to 10 mm. Enlargement of a colonic

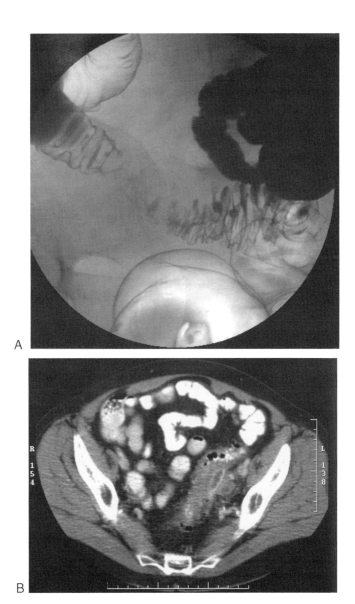

FIGURE 2.3.1.4.1A,B. Diverticular disease. (A) Double contrast barium enema (DCBE) demonstrates a typical diverticular stricture likely to be associated with a diverticular abscess. (B) Axial CT image of the pelvis (3 months later) demonstrating sigmoid diverticulitis and confirming the presence of an intramural abscess with avid wall enhancement.

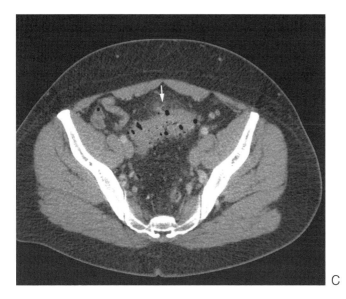

C

FIGURE 2.3.1.4.1C. Diverticular disease. Axial CECT image of sigmoid diverticulitis (arrow) in a different patient without evidence of stenosis or perforation.

diverticulum leads to stretching of the vasa recta located at the dome of the lesion. Weakening and erosions into those vessels leads to intraluminal bleeding. The hemorrhage tends to be significant and of arterial source.

It is important to appreciate from both imaging and management point of view that diverticular disease represents a spectrum of stages:

- Prediverticular stage: manifested by thickening of colonic wall and the presence of immature diverticula.
- Diverticulosis stage: well-formed diverticula.
- Diverticulitis: localized pericolic inflammation leading to small abscesses due to diverticula perforation and/or stricture formation.

CT with oral/rectal and intravenous contrast medium is the imaging modality of choice, especially in the diverticulitis phase. CT is excellent in diagnosing complications of diverticulitis such as perforation, intraabdominal collections, fistulae, portal vein thrombosis, and liver abscesses.

---

## CT Features in Acute Diverticulitis

- Small colonic outpouching filled with air/contrast medium
- Colonic wall thickening with marked enhancement
- *Arrowhead* sign: edema at the orifice of inflamed diverticulum
- Stranding of the pericolic fat, fascial thickening
- Pericolic changes such as abscess and/or sinus formation, colovesical fistulas
- Free intraabdominal air and/or fluid
- Thrombus within the superior mesenteric/portal vein
- Liver abscesses

---

Double-contrast barium enema is a traditional imaging test. In diverticulosis stage, it clearly shows multiple diverticula as flask-like protrusions with broad necks (in profile) or ring shadows of well-circumscribed barium collections—*bowler hat* sign (en face). If acute diverticulitis or perforation is suspected, water-soluble contrast medium is used. Findings include:

- Marked thickening and distortion of haustral folds.
- Focal area of asymmetric narrowing of the bowel lumen caused by intramural inflammation and mucosal tethering.
- Longitudinal intramural fistulous tracts (*double tracking*).
- Fistulas to bladder, vagina, or small bowel.
- Pericolonic abscesses.
- Strictures, especially in the sigmoid colon. These can be difficult to distinguish from malignant strictures and sometimes cause large bowel obstruction.

There is little place for plain radiography, apart from demonstrating complications such as perforation and big diverticular abscesses. In those cases, plain abdominal X-ray can demonstrate signs of pneumoperitoneum or mottled gas collection outside the bowel, more commonly around the sigmoid in cases of abscess formation. Air within the bladder is seen with colovesical fistulas.

*2.3.1.4.2 Colorectal Carcinoma* Colorectal cancer is the most common malignancy of the GI tract and the third most common cancer overall. The majority (65%) occur in rectum and sigmoid colon and 98% are adenocarcinomas on histopathology. Colorectal neoplasms account for approximately 5% of significant lower GI bleeding. Double-contrast barium enema is an excellent imaging modality for the diagnosis of colorectal cancer but is being supplanted by CT colonography (CTC). In this procedure, the colon is cleansed as for a barium enema or colonoscopy and it is then distended with air prior to imaging. The images can either be viewed in two-dimensional format or reconstructed into three-dimensional virtual imaging format, or "fly through." This is a particularly sensitive test for demonstrating adenomatous polyps that are the precursor for colorectal cancer, and it rivals optical colonoscopy in their detection. Frank carcinomas are demonstrated as polypoid masses, circumferential thickening of the bowel wall, or as a malignant stricture. Other changes include stranding of the pericolic fat, tumor extension through the bowel wall or into adjacent organs, lymphadenopathy, and liver metastasis.

Barium enema if performed shows colorectal cancer as either an anular or polypoid lesion. Annular or *apple core* lesions are usually found in the sigmoid colon. They appear as circumferential narrowing of the bowel with shouldering and mucosal destruction. They also can result in large bowel obstruction. Polypoid lesions are usually large and are more commonly found in rectum or cecum, shown as large filling defects.

MR has a particular role in the local staging of rectal cancers and their relationships to the mesorectal fascia. This is relevant to the need or otherwise for neoadjuvant treatment.

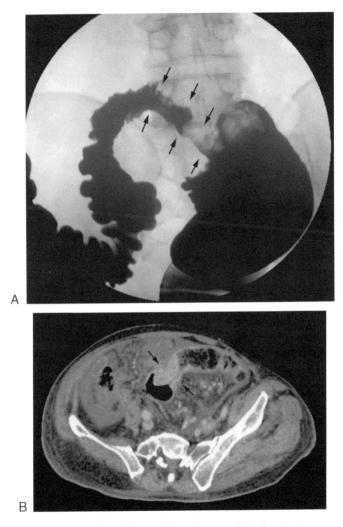

FIGURE 2.3.1.4.2A,B. Colorectal carcinoma. (A) Contrast enema demonstrates an *apple core* lesion (arrows) in the rectosigmoid junction in keeping with a carcinoma. (B) CECT confirms the presence of the tumor (arrows) and shows a mild degree of distal large bowel obstruction and ascites.

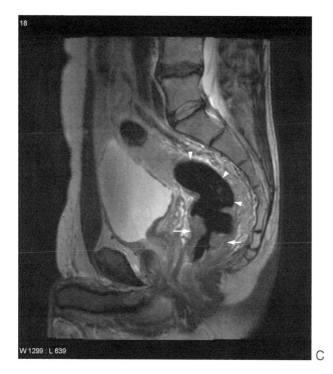

C

FIGURE 2.3.1.4.2C. Colorectal carcinoma. Sagittal T2-weighted MRI image of rectal cancer (arrows). The presence of negative contrast agent (arrowheads) in the rectal lumen increases the accuracy of local staging.

*2.3.1.4.3 Inflammatory Bowel Disease* Low GI bleeding typically occurs with ulcerative colitis (UC), but sometimes ileocolic Crohn's disease can present with profuse rectal bleeding due to arterial perforation.

Ulcerative colitis is a chronic diffuse inflammatory disease that involves the colorectal mucosa. Inflammation is limited to mucosa and submucosa, whereas in Crohn's disease, there is transmural involvement. It usually begins in the rectum and may progress proximally to involve the whole colon. In 30% of the patients, there is involvement of the terminal ileum (backwash ileitis). Patients with ulcerative colitis have an increased risk of developing colorectal cancer, especially

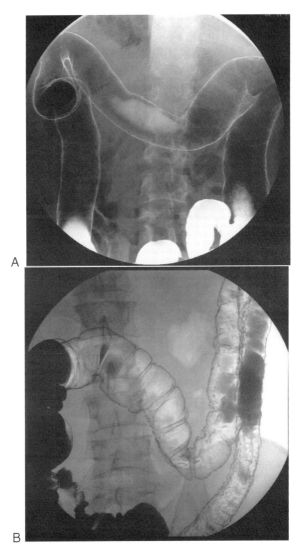

FIGURE 2.3.1.4.3A,B. (A) Ulcerative colitis. DCBE demonstrates an ahaustral colon with fine granular background - typical appearances of ulcerative colitis. Also note the gaping ileocecal valve (prone image). (B) Crohn's disease. DCBE demonstrates typical appearances of Crohn's disease with discrete asymmetrical ulceration and skip lesions.

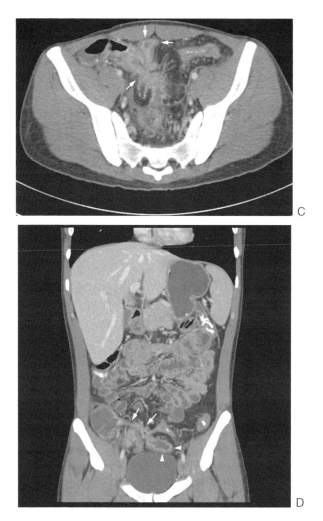

FIGURE 2.3.1.4.3C,D. Crohn's disease. (C) Axial CECT of a complex ileal-cecal fistula with thickening and increased enhancement of the ileal wall (arrows). (D) Coronal reformatted image demonstrating the complex fistula (arrows) and thickened ileal wall (arrowheads).

in the case of pancolitis where 75% of the patients develop colorectal cancer.

Double-contrast barium enema is an excellent diagnostic test. Imaging findings depend on the phase of the disease.

---

# Barium Enema Findings in Ulcerative Colitis

Acute phase

- Fine granular pattern of colonic mucosa
- *Collar button* ulcers
- Edematous, thickened haustra
- Inflammatory pseudopolyps
- Narrowing of the colorectal lumen

Chronic phase

- Rigidity and symmetric narrowing of the colonic lumen giving the appearances of *lead-pipe* colon
- Loss of haustrations and shortening of the colon
- Inflammation of the terminal ileum (backwash ileitis)
- Widening of the presacral space more than 1.5 cm
- Benign colonic strictures

---

CT features of UC are nonspecific and can be very difficult to differentiate from other colitides, especially Crohn's disease, based on imaging features alone. CT demonstrates narrowing of the large bowel lumen caused by diffuse, symmetrical thickening of colonic wall, which is less marked than in Crohn's disease. It shows widening of the presacral space due to proliferation of perirectal fat. Contrast-enhanced CT demonstrates the *target* or *halo* sign, which is the same as that in Crohn's disease. Other features include enhancement of inflammatory pseudopolyps and stranding of the pericolic fat.

Crohn's disease is a chronic granulomatous inflammatory bowel disease. It can occur anywhere in the bowel from the mouth to the anus but most frequently affects the terminal ileum and proximal large bowel. Barium follow-through/enteroclysis and CT are very good in the diagnosis of the disease and its complications, and MRI is sensitive in detecting fistulas and sinuses that can be difficult to appreciate on other imaging modalities.

---

## Barium Studies Findings in Crohn's Disease

- Skip lesions: affected and normal intervening areas
- Asymmetrical thickening of the bowel all due to a combination of inflammation and fibrosis
- Aphthoid ulcers: punctate barium collections surrounded by a halo
- Fissuring ulcers
- Cobblestone pattern: combination of longitudinal and transverse ulcers
- Sacculations on the antimesenteric side of the bowel
- Inflammatory pseudopolyps
- Luminal narrowing and multiple strictures especially involving terminal ileum (*string* sign)
- Sinus tracts, fistulas, and anorectal lesions

---

CT findings depend on the stage of the disease. In the acute stage, there is asymmetrical bowel wall thickening greater than 1 cm. A similar degree of thickening may be seen in pseudomembranous colitis. The *target* or *double-halo* sign on CECT is produced by intense enhancement of inner mucosa and outer muscularis propria layers, whereas edematous thickened submucosa is of low attenuation. In the chronic stage, there is luminal narrowing and reduced attenuation of thickened bowel wall indicating irreversible transmural fibrosis. CT can elegantly demonstrate mesenteric changes such as stranding of the mesenteric fat and low-volume mesenteric lymphadenopathy. CT is also useful in the diagnosis of disease complications such as abscesses and fistulas.

MRI examination using T2W fat-suppressed imaging or T1W imaging with intravenous Gd-DTPA are excellent for detecting and mapping fistulas, sinuses, and abscesses especially in perianal Crohn's disease. Transrectal US can be useful particularly in the evaluation of the anal sphincter in cases of anal involvement.

*2.3.1.4.4 Meckel's Diverticulum*   Meckel's diverticulum is a congenital true diverticulum of the ileum. It occurs in the antimesenteric border of the distal ileum, approximately 60 cm proximal to the ileocecal valve. Meckel's diverticulum usually contains ileal mucosa, but it can contain ectopic tissue, such as gastric or pancreatic mucosa, in up to 50%. Bleeding is rare, but when it occurs, it is associated with the presence of gastric mucosa. Hemorrhage is usually seen in children and is very rare in young adults.

Angiography is the best imaging test in setting of acute hemorrhage. It shows extravasation of contrast medium into the diverticulum and elegantly demonstrates the persistent vitello-intestinal artery as a long, nonbranching vessel arising from a distal ileal artery. Scintigraphy using $^{99m}$Tc pertechnetate is a well-recognized technique for identifying a Meckel's diverticulum that contains ectopic gastric mucosa. The area of ectopic uptake is seen within 5 to 10 minutes of radionuclide injection as an area of increase tracer uptake in the lower abdomen, usually on the right side. The overall diagnostic accuracy is low as the test is positive only in those diverticula that contain ectopic gastric mucosa. Small bowel enema (enteroclysis) may be performed when the diagnosis of Meckel's diverticulum is suspected. It is a more reliable technique than barium follow-through. The diverticulum appears as a blind-ending sac arising from the antimesenteric border of the distal ileum. Occasionally, the diverticulum may invert appearing as a filling defect, which may sometimes become the leading point of an intussusception.

*2.3.1.4.5 Angiodysplasia*  Angiodysplasia represents vascular ectasia in microcirculation of the mucous and the submucous layers of the bowel and occurs primarily in

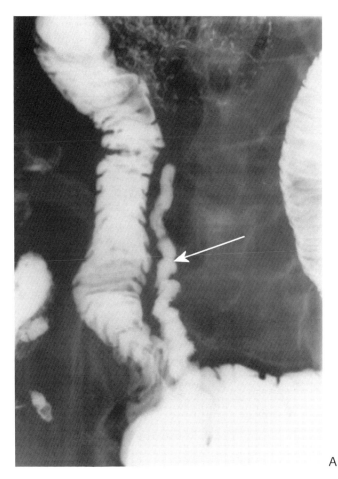

A

FIGURE 2.3.1.4.4A. Meckel's diverticulum. Barium follow through examination showing a blind ending sac (arrow) arising from the antimesenteric border of distal ileum. (*Continued*)

the ascending colon and cecum in middle-age and elderly patients. It is the most common cause of occult lower GI hemorrhage, but massive bleeding is very uncommon. Angiography is the imaging test of choice with excellent results when performed during a bleeding episode. It

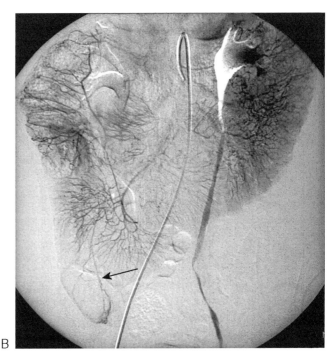

B

FIGURE 2.3.1.4.4B. (*Continued*) Meckel's diverticulum. Angiogram in a different patient shows persistent vitello-intestinal artery (arrow) as a long nonbranching vessel arising from a distal ileal artery.

demonstrates one or more tiny lakes of contrast medium on the antimesenteric border of the bowel. In addition, early-filling veins may be seen draining the abnormal area.

## 2.3.2 Hematuria

Hematuria can be the presenting symptom of a variety of renal tract pathologies including stone disease, infection, neoplasms, and trauma. Diagnostic imaging of stone disease and transitional cell carcinoma have been discussed in detail in Section 2.1.2.9, and imaging of renal trauma will be

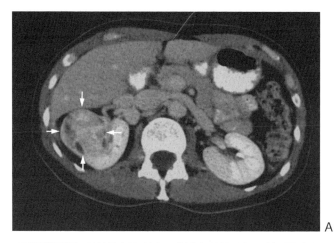

A

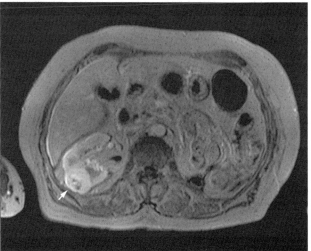

B

FIGURE 2.3.2A,B. Renal cell carcinoma. (A) CECT showing a heterogeneously enhancing mass (arrows) originating from the midportion of the right kidney in keeping with a renal cell carcinoma. (B) Axial T1-weighted image of the arterial phase of a contrast-enhanced MRI (different patient) showing a right-sided RCC (arrow) as strongly enhancing mass.

discussed in Section 2.5.2. A general view of the best diagnostic approach in patients with hematuria is given in this section. Imaging features of renal cell carcinoma are also described.

A combination of US and cystoscopy remains the best screening test for hematuria. US is more sensitive than IVU in demonstrating small renal masses situated outside the collecting system. A hematuria service, with early clinical examination, urine cytology testing, and US, is frequently provided for painless hematuria in many centers. IVU provides good anatomic definition of the kidneys and, to some extent, an indication of their function. It is especially sensitive in the detection of small endothelial lesions. CT is excellent for diagnosis and staging of renal cell carcinoma.

*Renal cell carcinoma (RCC)* is the most common primary renal tumor. Gross hematuria is the most common presenting symptom (60%). However, more than 50% of RCCs are incidentally found on CT, US, or MRI of the abdomen. US demonstrates a hyperechoic, hypoechoic, or in the majority of cases an isoechoic mass. Cystic RCCs typically have multiple thickened septae and nodular solid components. Color Doppler US is useful in detecting tumor thrombus extension to the renal vein and IVC.

At CT and on unenhanced images, RCC appears as a soft tissue mass that contains calcifications in up to 30% of the cases. Multiphase CT imaging is ideal for staging and preoperative planning of RCC. Most RCCs are hypervascular on contrast-enhanced CT images. They are best seen on nephrographic phase (renal enhancement at capillary level) images, whereas small intrarenal RCC can be missed on corticomedullary phase (enhancing renal cortex with limited medullary enhancement). Contrast-enhanced CT is very accurate for detecting tumor extension to the IVC and renal vein, as well as distant metastasis such as liver, adrenal, lung, bone, and so forth. Three-dimensional CT reconstruction with volume rendering and maximum projection techniques are excellent for preoperative staging, and MRI can provide additional information on vascular involvement if required.

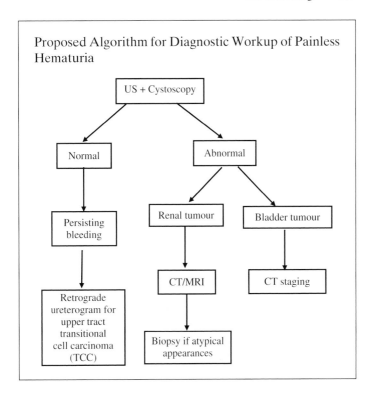

Proposed Algorithm for Diagnostic Workup of Painless Hematuria

US + Cystoscopy

Normal

Abnormal

Persisting bleeding

Renal tumour

Bladder tumour

Retrograde ureterogram for upper tract transitional cell carcinoma (TCC)

CT/MRI

CT staging

Biopsy if atypical appearances

## *Suggestions for Further Reading*

1. Chen CY, Wu DC, Kang WY, Hsu JS. Staging of gastric cancer with 16 channel-MDCT. Abdom Imaging 2006;31: 514–520.

2. Low VHS. Diagnosis of gastric carcinoma: sensitivity of double-contrast barium studies. AJR 1994;162:329–334.

3. Miettinen M, El-Rifai W, Sobin L, Lasota J. Evaluation of malignancy and prognosis of gastrointestinal stromal tumours: a review. Hum Pathol 2002;33:478–483.

4. Howarth DM. The role of nuclear medicine in the detection of acute gastrointestinal bleeding. Semin Nucl Med 2006;36(2): 133–146.

5. Browder W, Cerise EJ, Litwin MS. Impact of emergency angiography in massive lower gastrointestinal bleeding. Ann Surg 1986;204:530.

6. Gore RM, Miller FH, Pereles FS, Yaghmai V, Berlin JW. Helical CT in the evaluation of the acute abdomen. AJR 2000;174: 901–913.

# 2.4 Jaundice

*Jaundice*, a yellow pigmentation of the skin, mucous membranes, and sclera, results from excess circulating bilirubin. It is usually described as prehepatic, hepatic, or posthepatic but only the latter, essentially mechanical biliary obstruction is amenable to surgical treatment, and this will be discussed.

## *2.4.1 Radiologic Evaluation of Mechanical Biliary Obstruction*

The two major causes of bile duct obstruction are biliary stones and malignant tumors. Stone disease is the most common followed by carcinoma of the head of the pancreas. Other tumors include ampullary tumors, cholangiocarcinoma, gallbladder carcinoma, and porta hepatis lymphadenopathy. Benign biliary strictures resulting from acute pancreatitis may also cause biliary obstruction, as may ischemia.

The combination of clinical assessment and radiologic examination provides an accurate diagnosis of the cause of posthepatic jaundice in 98% of patients. Plain abdominal radiographs are usually unhelpful in the assessment of patients presenting with jaundice. They may show calcified biliary stones in 10% of the patients, and pancreatic area calcification is suggestive of chronic pancreatitis.

The diagnosis of extrahepatic and/or intrahepatic bile duct dilatation is a crucial step in the evaluation of the jaundiced patient. US is used as the primary imaging technique to diagnose the presence of duct dilatation and distinguish between obstructive and nonobstructive jaundice. Dilated intrahepatic bile ducts appear as branching hypoechoic structures radiating from the porta hepatis, paralleling the portal vein and hepatic arterial branches but with no flow within. They are often detected first in the left lobe of the liver. US can define the site and cause of biliary obstruction in only 30% of cases as the lower common bile duct is often obscured by overlying bowel gas. Where US is equivocal for the presence of bile duct dilatation or is unable to identify the underlying etiology, magnetic resonance cholangiopancreatography (MRCP) is used as this is unaffected by bowel gas.

In a patient where biliary obstruction has been diagnosed by US, and gallstones are demonstrated convincingly as the cause, endoscopic retrograde cholangiopancreatography (ERCP) should be the next investigation. It can reliably demonstrate the dilated biliary system, confirm the presence of calculi, and allow their extraction after sphincterotomy.

Where the initial investigations indicate biliary duct obstruction due to a likely malignant cause, the ideal next step is to stage the tumor in order to assess the operability. This is best performed with CECT, prior to any drainage procedure, allowing demonstration of an obstructing mass and staging-related information such as local nodal enlargement and vascular invasion. Additional information can be provided using both MRI, endoscopic ultrasound, and ERCP where appropriate. At ERCP, plastic or self-expandable metal stents can also be placed to relieve the jaundice.

Percutaneous transhepatic cholangiography (PTC) is less frequently used in the assessment of obstructive jaundice but is valuable where palliative drainage is required and where ERCP has failed. Typically, this is in patients with extensive hilar malignancy, benign biliary strictures, or after gastroduodenal surgery.

Nuclear medicine studies using $^{99m}$Tc-labeled N-substituted iminodiacetic acid compounds ($^{99m}$Tc-HIDA) have no role in imaging of obstructive jaundice because of impaired bilirubin excretion but are useful in the evaluation of low-grade obstruction, after bile duct surgery, and so forth.

Suggested Algorithm in Diagnosis of Obstructive Jaundice

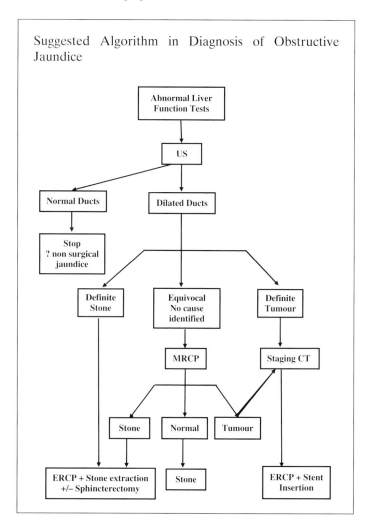

## 2.4.1.1 Biliary Stones

Gallstones are present in approximately 15% of the adult population in the United Kingdom. There are three common types of gallstones: cholesterol, pigmented, and mixed stones.

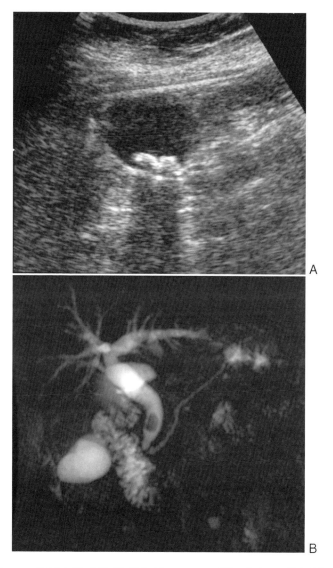

FIGURE 2.4.1A,B. (A) Gallbladder stones. US of the gallbladder demonstrating two echogenic foci within the gallbladder representing gallbladder stones. (B) Common bile duct stones. MRCP image demonstrating a well-defined low-signal-intensity filling defect within the common bile duct representing a stone.

US is more than 95% accurate in the diagnosis of gallstones in the gallbladder. They appear as one or more hyperechoic foci with related acoustic shadowing. They change position with change in patient position. US can also reliably assess the presence of associated inflammatory changes in the gallbladder.

Approximately 15% of patients with gallstones have stones within the bile ducts that may appear as hyperechoic foci within the common bile duct, which is usually dilated. The normal range of US measurements for the diameter of the common hepatic duct is commonly accepted as up to 6 mm, unless there has been a cholecystectomy in which case 10 mm is considered the upper limit of normal. The bile duct should be measured where the right main hepatic artery crosses the common hepatic duct. The sensitivity of US in detecting choledocholithiasis is poor, and compared with ERCP, US is only 20% to 30% accurate in the diagnosis of the common bile duct calculi. This is due to several factors including normal-caliber ducts and obscuring of ducts by overlying bowel gas. MRCP is much more accurate, and endoscopic US can improve accuracy further for detecting small distal common bile duct stones.

ERCP is the next step if US confirms bile duct stones or if there is a strong clinical suspicion of duct stones but equivocal US findings. ERCP has the major advantage of endoscopic sphincterotomy and stone removal, which does not necessitate any further treatment in the elderly population, whereas younger patients are referred for subsequent cholecystectomy. If there is doubt about the diagnosis MRCP is next indicated as a noninvasive diagnostic test. ERCP should be reserved in most cases for its therapeutic potential.

## 2.4.1.2 Carcinoma of the Head of the Pancreas

Ductal adenocarcinoma of the pancreatic head is the most common malignant cause of obstructive jaundice. US shows a dilated common bile duct with abrupt termination at the level of the pancreatic head. It may demonstrate a hypoechoic mass at the head of the pancreas as well as local lymphadenopathy and liver metastasis. It is not a sensitive technique for detecting small lesions.

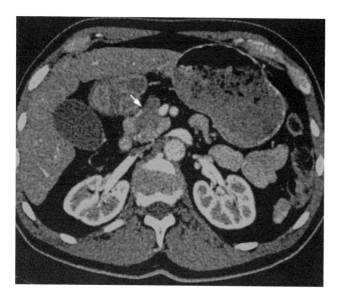

FIGURE 2.4.1. Carcinoma of the head of the pancreas. Arterial phase CECT of the abdomen showing a low-attenuation lesion (arrow) within the normal enhancing pancreatic head representing a pancreatic carcinoma.

CECT, as described in detail in Section 2.2.1.3, is the technique of choice for both diagnosis and staging of the disease. The tumor appears as a low-attenuation lesion within the head of normal avidly enhancing pancreas (best seen in arterial and pancreatic phases). Local tumor extension into porta hepatis structures such as the portal vein and contiguous invasion into the adjacent duodenum, stomach, and mesentery can be demonstrated.

ERCP demonstrates significant dilation of common bile duct with irregular distal *rat-tail* stricture and prestenotic dilatation. As the majority of the cases are inoperable, it is usually the practice to place a bile duct stent for palliative purposes.

## 2.4.1.3 Tumors of the Biliary Tract

These include cholangiocarcinoma, ampullary carcinoma, and carcinoma of the gallbladder.

*Cholangiocarcinoma* is a malignant tumor that arises from the epithelium of intra- or extrahepatic bile ducts. It is the second most common primary malignant liver tumor after hepatocellular carcinoma. It may arise from any part of the biliary tree, but a specific subtype involving the confluence of right and left hepatic ducts is referred to as a Klatskin tumor. Imaging is often challenging, as the tumor volume may be small, and best achieved by a combination of techniques such as CECT, MRI, and if needed ERCP/PTC.

US may show a heterogeneous, hypoechoic mass with intrahepatic duct dilatation or dilatation of both intra- and extrahepatic ducts in common bile duct lesions. CECT with three phases of enhancement—arterial, portal, and delayed phase—is the best imaging test with a very good sensitivity especially for large lesions. Gadolinium-enhanced T1W MRI and multislice CECT are probably equivalent for detecting small hilar tumors, as well as intrahepatic disease extension and periductal tumor infiltration.

---

## CT findings in cholangiocarcinoma

Nonenhanced CT

- Low attenuation single/multiple lesions at the periphery, or central at the confluence of the ductal system, or at the level of common bile duct with intrahepatic bile duct dilatation

Arterial phase (at 35 seconds postinjection)

- Early rim-enhancement with heterogeneous central enhancement of the lesion

Portal phase (at 70 seconds postinjection)

- Less marked enhancement of the lesion

Delayed phase (at 10 minutes postinjection)

- Persistent enhancing tumor (more than the adjacent liver) due to fibrous stroma

ERCP is a valuable imaging technique permitting diagnostic biopsy and palliative intervention procedures. ERCP findings include:

- Multiple long concentric strictures of intrahepatic ducts with associated diffuse prestenotic dilatation
- Ductal wall irregularity
- Hilar strictures with associated proximal intrahepatic bile duct dilatation in Klatskin tumors
- Intraductal lobulated filling defect in common bile duct tumors

In the event of a failed ERCP, PTC may be performed. *Ampullary carcinoma* is a malignant tumor arising from the ampulla of Vater. CECT with duodenal distension with water is the best imaging modality for diagnosis and staging of the disease. It demonstrates a hypodense, lobulated soft tissue mass at the ampulla. There is also dilatation of both common bile duct and pancreatic duct (the *double-duct* sign). ERCP shows intra- and extrahepatic bile duct dilatation, and dilated common duct coming to an abrupt end often with significant shouldering, suggestive of malignancy. Concomitant biopsies can also be taken at the time of ERCP as the ampulla itself frequently appears abnormal, although frequently much of the tumor is submucosal. On gadolinium-enhanced T1W MRI, adenocarcinoma of the ampulla appears as a hypointense lesion compared with high-signal normal enhancing pancreatic tissue. MRCP will show similar appearances to ERCP.

*Gallbladder carcinoma* it is the fifth most common GI malignancy. It usually presents as a large soft tissue mass infiltrating the gallbladder fossa and carries a very poor prognosis. Plain abdominal radiograph is often noncontributory, though it may show presence of calcified gallstones and porcelain gallbladder, both predisposing conditions for gallbladder carcinoma. US findings include a hypoechoic mass infiltrating the gallbladder fossa, irregular diffuse thickening of the gallbladder wall, echogenic mucosal polypoid mass larger than 1 cm, gallstones, and occasionally a calcified *porcelain* gallbladder wall. CECT demonstrates a hypovascular mass infiltrating the gallbladder fossa with presence of gallstones or porcelain gallbladder. It often shows tumor extension into the adjacent liver and porta hepatis. MRI is rarely performed in practice as a combination of US and CT usually provides an accurate diagnosis in most patients.

## Suggestions for Further Reading

1. Han JK, Choi BI, Kim AY, et al. Cholangiocarcinoma: pictorial essay of CT and cholangiographic findings. Radiographics 2002;22:173–187.
2. Talamini MA, Moesinger RC, Pitt HA, et al. Adenocarcinoma of the ampulla of Vater. Ann Surg 1997;225:590–600.
3. Levy AD, Murakata LA, Rohrmann CA Jr. Gallbladder carcinoma: radiologic-pathologic correlation. Radiographics 2001;21:295–314.
4. Ichikawa T, Erturk SM, Sou H, et al. MDCT of pancreatic adenocarcinoma: optimal imaging phases and multiplanar reformatted imaging. AJR Am J Roentgenol 2006;187(6):1513–1520.
5. Slattery JM, Sahani DV. What is the current state-of-the-art imaging for detection and staging of cholangiocarcinoma? Oncologist 2006;11(8):913–922.

## 2.5 Trauma

Imaging plays a crucial role in the diagnosis and management of patients with trauma with CT the investigation of choice. New-generation multislice CT machines provide a very fast and robust data acquisition, completing examinations in a few minutes, which is very important in critically ill patients. The possibility of multiplanar reconstruction is helpful in planning complicated surgical interventions in patients with multiorgan trauma, particularly skeletal. It goes without saying that an early competent clinical assessment is important to ensure that imaging studies cover all the relevant body organs at risk.

## 2.5.1 Chest Trauma

Major chest trauma rarely occurs in isolation and is usually part of polytrauma. Head injury, fractures of the

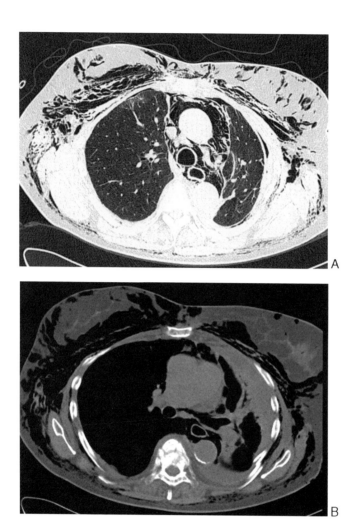

FIGURE 2.5.1A,B. Chest trauma. CT of the chest at (A) lung and (B) bone windows showing significant pneumomediastinum, pneumopericardium, as well as extensive surgical emphysema within the soft tissues of the anterior thoracic wall. Note posterior left rib and vertebral body fractures.

vertebral column and extremities, and abdominal and pelvic trauma are all common associated injuries. One or several thoracic structures or organs can be damaged due to blunt or penetrating chest trauma. This can lead to thoracic cage fractures, pneumothorax and hemothorax, pulmonary contusion, diaphragmatic rupture, pneumomediastinum, and aortic dissection/rupture. Although plain chest radiograph is usually the first imaging performed in a patient with suspected chest trauma, most patients will proceed to CT.

Plain chest radiograph will demonstrate only 50% of rib fractures. Extensive views looking for subtle rib fractures are not indicated in the acute situation. They do not alter a patient's management as they are almost always treated conservatively. It is more important to detect associated injuries and complications such as pneumothorax or pulmonary contusions. Imaging findings in pneumothorax are described in Section 2.1.1.1. Lung contusion occurs in the majority of cases of blunt chest trauma. Contusions appear as areas of peripheral consolidation, usually adjacent to the ribs or spine. Changes on the chest radiograph appear within 6 hours of trauma and persist for up to a week. Nonresolving or progressing areas of consolidations should raise the suspicion of adult respiratory distress syndrome (ARDS) or fat embolism.

Fractures of the upper three ribs imply severe trauma that may have resulted in damage to the great vessels, brachial plexus, spinal or major airways. Fractures of the lower three ribs raise suspicion for associated injuries to spleen, liver, and kidneys, and further imaging of the abdomen should be performed. In children, rib fractures are rare as accidental injuries, and their presence should alert those responsible for the management of the patient to nonaccidental injury. Sternal fractures occur less frequently than rib fractures but they carry a relatively high mortality due to associated mediastinal injuries. Lateral sternal views can reliably diagnose sternal fractures, and CT can elegantly demonstrate associated injuries. Thoracic spine fractures are often overlooked on the initial assessment especially if there are no neurologic signs. CT demonstrates the presence of the fracture as well as other features such as paraspinal hematoma, spinal cord contusion, and so forth.

Hemothorax is frequently present in patients with chest trauma. It usually produces a meniscus sign on a conventional erect chest radiograph (CXR). However, in trauma patients, it is likely that the CXR is taken in a supine position and therefore the blood tracks posterior to the lungs producing a diffuse increased opacification of the affected hemithorax rather than classic meniscus sign. If CXR findings are equivocal, then CT is indicated.

Pneumomediastinum is usually caused by tracheobronchial or esophageal ruptures. The CXR appearances are of vertical lucencies that outline mediastinal structures, especially on the left side, and often extend into the neck and/or chest wall. These features are better appreciated on a lateral CXR. CT is more sensitive than plain radiography in demonstrating the presence and extent of the pneumomediastinum. Bronchial tears are uncommon, and the majority occur in the main stem bronchus. They are usually associated with other extensive injuries such as fractures of the upper ribs, sternum, and thoracic spine. CXR demonstrates the presence of pneumothorax, pneumomediastinum, and the *fallen lung* sign with complete rupture. CT with coronal reconstruction is more sensitive in locating the site of the tear and demonstrating associated injuries.

Traumatic aortic rupture due to rapid deceleration at impact causes 15% to 20% of road traffic accident deaths. The majority of those surviving an aortic rupture have ruptures at the isthmus, just distal to the origin of the left subclavian artery where the aorta is most fixed. The initial radiologic evaluation is likely to be a CXR, which will be abnormal in 70% of the patients. Aortic rupture is a surgical emergency that requires prompt diagnosis and surgical repair in virtually all cases.

---

## Plain Chest Radiographs Findings in Aortic Rupture

- Widening of the superior mediastinum (more than 8 cm or more than 25% of thoracic width)

- Loss of definition of the aortic knuckle
- Depression of the left main bronchus
- Displacement of the trachea and the nasogastric tube to the right
- Left apical pleural cap and left pleural effusion
- Associated fractures of the upper three ribs

CT is the next imaging test performed in suspected aortic rupture if the patient is hemodynamically stable. It elegantly demonstrates direct signs of aortic rupture such as intimal flap, irregularity of the aortic contour, and pseudoaneurysms, as well as indirect signs of hemomediastinum. It is very important to obtain unenhanced images first in order to confirm the presence of fresh blood. Reformatted CT images have a very high sensitivity and specificity for diagnosing aortic rupture; however, an unexplained hemomediastinum may require urgent catheter angiography

Diaphragmatic rupture occurs in less than 5% of patients with significant blunt thoracoabdominal trauma. Tears are usually at least 10 cm long, radially oriented, and usually occur at the weakest part of the diaphragm—the posterior aspect of the musculo-tendinous junction. Left- and right-sided tears occur with equal frequencies but left-sided ones are diagnosed easier than the right-sided tears, the majority of which are missed. This is due to the fact that liver herniation through a right-sided tear retains the smooth contour of the hemidiaphragm, which is interpreted mistakenly as normal on a CXR. Prompt diagnosis of diaphragmatic rupture is very important because surgical repair of the tear is mandatory, as they do not heal spontaneously.

As noted, the CXR is insensitive in the diagnosis of diaphragmatic rupture, being abnormal in less than 50% of the cases. Radiographic findings may include:

- Elevation of the hemidiaphragm (comparison with old films is very important)
- Loss of the diaphragmatic contour

- Contralateral mediastinal shift
- Presence of hollow viscera within the thorax
- Coiled nasogastric tube within the left hemithorax

CT is the best available technique, though it is sometimes difficult to visualize the dome of the diaphragm as it usually lies tangential to the axial plane. Multislice CT with its ability to produce coronal and sagittal reformatted images has significantly improved the sensitivity and specificity of CT. Features of diaphragmatic rupture on CT include interruption of normal diaphragmatic contour, and herniation of the abdominal contents within the chest. On the left side, this results in the *collar* sign (constriction of the stomach as it passes through the tear into the chest) and on the right side the *cottage loaf* sign with the liver herniating through the diaphragm. US is very good in visualizing the diaphragm especially if outlined by fluid and can reliably diagnose tears. The examination is difficult if the patient is very tender or if there are complications such as extensive surgical emphysema, pneumothorax, and so forth, which will impair visualization of the diaphragm. These factors together with its operator dependence limit the role of US in routine imaging of the diaphragmatic rupture. MRI is excellent in detecting diaphragmatic tears, although its use in practice is limited because of MRI incompatibility of some life-support devices used in trauma patients. Direct multiplanar imaging is very important in detecting small tears. They are best shown in T1W sequence where the diaphragm appears as a low-intensity line outlined on either sides by high-intensity mediastinal and abdominal fat.

## 2.5.2 Abdominal Trauma

Abdominopelvic trauma accounts for a large proportion of morbidity and mortality in multitrauma patients. Multiple life-threatening injuries often coexist, requiring rapid triage with simultaneous diagnostic and therapeutic interventions. The choice of imaging modalities depends to a large extent on local availability and expertise. In practice, CECT is the

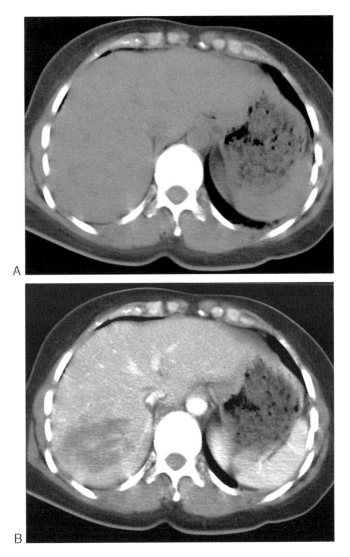

FIGURE 2.5.2A,B. Liver trauma. (A) Unenhanced and (B) portal phase CECT of the abdomen demonstrating an irregular low-attenuation area in the posterior aspect of the right lobe of the liver (best appreciated on the CECT image) representing liver laceration.

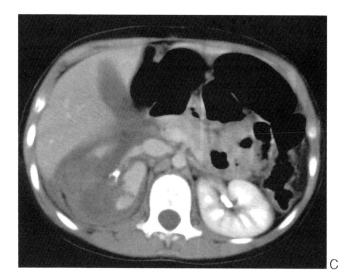

FIGURE 2.5.2C. Kidney trauma. CECT of the abdomen showing lack of perfusion in the posterior aspect of the right kidney. Note also the presence of free perirenal fluid in this trauma patient.

most useful and quickest method. Imaging findings in liver, pancreatic, splenic, and urinary tract trauma are described in this section.

## 2.5.2.1 Hepatic Trauma

The liver is the most frequently injured intraabdominal organ. Trauma to the liver can lead to parenchymal laceration, capsular rupture, intraparenchymal or subcapsular hematoma. Laceration may involve major vessels and can lead to massive hemorrhage. Imaging plays a crucial role in hepatic trauma except when patients require immediate surgery because of extensive life-threatening injuries. At CT examination, initial unenhanced images are mandatory in order to demonstrate high-attenuation fresh hemorrhage. The location of fresh clot can be a good indication of a nearby site and source of bleeding. Postcontrast images are also mandatory when organ trauma is suspected. Portal phase images are excellent in detecting subtle lacerations of the liver, and arterial phase images should be performed to indicate hepatic artery trauma when an injury involving the porta is suspected. US can reliably demonstrate the presence of free intraabdominal fluid, suggesting liver laceration or capsular rupture, but is not reliable for parenchymal tears. It is a very useful technique for the follow-up of the known lesions such as subcapsular hematomas as they resolve and for diagnosing complications such as intraabdominal collections. Angiography is only indicated in cases of continuing significant bleeding suggesting a vessel laceration. It reliably demonstrates the source of bleeding and guides therapeutic procedures such as embolization, thus avoiding open surgery.

## 2.5.2.2 Pancreatic Trauma

Pancreatic trauma is rare and is usually associated with other visceral injuries, especially of the liver and duodenum. It is typically caused by significant direct impact such as from a steering wheel or a seatbelt injury resulting in the midline compression of the pancreas against the vertebral column. This may result in fracture of the gland or main pancreatic duct disruption, which carries a high complication rate. Thin-slice CT with fast bolus contrast injection (3 to 4 mL/s) and oral contrast medium is the best technique for imaging of pancreatic trauma. Imaging features include fluid in the lesser sac, thickening of the anterior renal fascia, stranding of the peripancreatic fat, focal enlargement of the pancreas, and intraparenchymal hematoma. CT can elegantly show a fracture line through the gland and separation of fracture fragments. ERCP may be required if a pancreatic duct injury is suspected.

## 2.5.2.3 Splenic Trauma

The spleen is the most common intraabdominal organ to require surgery after injury. The current trend is toward conservative management because of increased incidence of postsplenectomy sepsis. However, delayed rupture can occur in this situation. CECT will show altered contour to the spleen in subcapsular hematomas and low-attenuation areas in intraparenchymal hematomas. Parenchymal lacerations appear as hypodense irregular lines (areas of nonenhancement) separating more dense splenic fragments (areas of normal enhancement). Splenic fracture is seen as deep laceration extending from the capsule to the splenic hilum. US plays little role in imaging of acute splenic trauma but is a good technique for the follow-up of patients that have been managed conservatively.

### 2.5.2.4 Renal Tract Trauma

Renal injury is seen in just fewer than 10% of patients with blunt or penetrating abdominal trauma. The American Association for the Surgery of Trauma (AAST) has described a renal injury severity score that is based on surgical observations. AAST injury grade varies from grade I (renal contusion or subcapsular hematoma) to grade V (shattered kidney with renal vascular pedicle injury). Most renal injuries are minor (grade I and II) and are managed conservatively. The main role of imaging in renal trauma is to help in deciding whether the patient should be managed conservatively or surgically. CECT is the initial study of choice in renal trauma. Nephrographic and parenchymal phases are valuable in demonstrating perfusion, active bleeding, and extent of parenchymal injury, and excretory phase is very useful in assessing the integrity of the collecting system. CECT findings depend on the grade of the injury.

---

## CECT Grading of Renal Injuries

Grade I injury

- Intraparenchymal contusion/hematoma: ill-defined area of reduced attenuation relative to normal kidney (parenchymal phase)
- Subcapsular hematoma: round fluid collection of relatively high attenuation (clotted blood)

- Small linear lacerations with hematoma adjacent to them
- Subsegmental cortical infarct: wedge-shaped low-attenuation area

Grade II injury

- Deeper laceration through cortex extending to medulla: hypodense area in the nephrographic phase
- Contrast medium extravasation into the perinephric space during the excretory phase
- Segmental cortical infarct

Grade III injury

- Renal lacerations extending into collecting system, vascular injury (active arterial contrast extravasation)
- *Cortical rim* sign representing preserved capsular enhancement a reliable sign of subacute infarction
- *Shattered kidney* pathognomonic of renal artery thrombosis: lack of enhancement of entire injured kidney
- Perinephric hematoma, hemoperitoneum

Grade IV injury

- Fragmentation of the kidney with large perinephric hematoma compromising renal perfusion
- Avulsion of the renal pedicle
- Active bleeding and urine extravasation into the peritoneal cavity

US has a low sensitivity and a very low negative predictive value for the diagnosis of renal trauma and cannot provide any functional information about the injured kidney. It is, however, a useful technique for the follow-up of posttraumatic intrarenal or perirenal collections. Limited IVU (single radiograph), usually taken in the operating theater (once the patient is stable) can be helpful as it allows the visualization of both kidneys and reliably diagnoses most of the major renal injuries. The only role of angiography in renal trauma is to demonstrate the vascular anatomy prior to reconstructive surgery.

### 2.5.2.5 Bladder Trauma

The bladder is the most commonly injured organ after blunt pelvic trauma. The presence of a full bladder increases the likelihood of bladder injury in pelvic trauma. The spectrum of injury includes bladder contusion, interstitial injury, and intraperitoneal rupture, extraperitoneal rupture, or a combination of both. Intraperitoneal rupture is caused by direct trauma to the distended bladder and usually occurs at the dome of the bladder. It accounts for 15% of bladder injuries. Extraperitoneal rupture is usually caused by bony fragments from anterior pelvic arch fractures and is located at the base of the bladder. It accounts for 85% of significant bladder injuries. CT cystography has been shown to be very useful especially in imaging of extraperitoneal bladder ruptures as it also elegantly demonstrates multiple pelvic fractures and any other concomitant injuries. Cystography shows contrast medium extravasation in paracolic gutters and around the bowel loops in cases of intraperitoneal bladder rupture. Findings in extraperitoneal rupture include perivesical contrast medium extravasation producing a *flame-shape* urinary bladder and extravasation of contrast medium into the perineum, anterior abdominal wall, scrotum, and so forth.

## *Suggestions for Further Reading*

1. Dee P. The radiology of chest trauma. Radiol Clin North Am 1992;30:291–306.
2. Shackleton KL, Stewart ET, Taylor AJ. Traumatic diaphragmatic injuries: spectrum of radiographic findings. Radiographics 1998;18:49–59.

3. Lubner M, Menias C, Rucker C, et al. Blood in the belly: CT findings of hemoperitoneum. Radiographics 2007;27(1):109–125.
4. Shanmuganathan K, Mirvis SE, Boyd-Kranis R, Takada T, Scalea TM. Non-surgical management of blunt splenic injury: use of CT criteria to select patients for splenic arteriography and potential endovascular therapy. Radiology 2000;217:75–82.
5. Kawashima A, Sandler CM, Corl FM, et al. Imaging of renal trauma: a comprehensive review. Radiographics 2001;21: 557–574.
6. Vaccaro JP, Brody JM. CT cystography in the evaluation of major bladder trauma. Radiographics 2000;20:1373–1381.

# Index

Printed in the United States